My Donkeybody

Living with a Body that No Longer Obeys You

Michael Wenham

16
EasyRead Large

RHYW

Copyright Page from the Original Book

First published in the UK in 2008 by Monarch Books
(a publishing imprint of Lion Hudson plc),
Wilkinson House, Jordan Hill Road, Oxford OX2 8DR.
Tel: +44 (0)1865 302750 Fax: +44 (0)1865 302757
Email: monarch@lionhudson.com
www.lionhudson.com

ISBN: 978-1-85424-889-3 (UK)
ISBN: 978-0-8254-6295-5 (USA)

Reprinted 2010.

Distributed by:
UK: Marston Book Services Ltd, PO Box 269, Abingdon, Oxon OX14 4YN;
USA: Kregel Publications, PO Box 2607, Grand Rapids, Michigan 49501

Back cover picture: Bryan Wenham

This book has been printed on paper and board independently certified as having come from sustainable forests.

British Library Cataloguing Data
A catalogue record for this book is available from the British Library.

TABLE OF CONTENTS

'In this transparently honest account of his long journey with Motor Neurone Disease Michael Wenham draws us into a world of struggle, pain and fear where trust in God is tested to the utmost. His account leaves little untouched; big issues like euthanasia are not ducked; disability, embarrassment, kindness from strangers are all openly shared. His brilliant story-telling makes the book hard to put down; his gentle humour delights and warms the reader. But the author's humanity and faith hit you most, describing without pretence the reality of life lived before God. I love this book. I think you will too.' – **Elaine Storkey,** president of Tear Fund and broadcaster

'My Donkeybody is a beautifully-written, honest story about suffering and grace. As Michael's suffering increased so God's grace abounds. I have been profoundly humbled by knowing Michael and profoundly moved by his love and faithfulness to Christ through the pain. This book will help us understand more of what it means for "God's grace to be made perfect in weakness."' – **Simon Ponsonby,** writer and theologian

'The Christian faith joyfully proclaims an upside-down wisdom where the powerful are toppled from their throne and the humble lifted high. The wisdom of God has always been revealed through what the world considers weak and useless: a man dying on a cross. Michael Wenham's account of how he lives and ministers with a terrible degenerative illness is another chapter in this astonishing story. His story tells us what it is like when Christian faith encounters terminal illness. There are no glib answers, no false comfort, just a joyful, humbling, funny and very realistic account of what it's like. And because it is so real it is very inspiring. To read it is to be put in touch with the reality of human suffering and with the tenacity of Christian hope.' – **Rt Revd Stephen Cottrell,** Bishop of Reading

'For anyone, the diagnosis of Motor Neurone Disease is devastating enough, but when it affects your voice first and you are a vicar, it might seem that your calling is over. Not for Michael. In this book he demonstrates that with simple determination, faith and support, life can be lived with MND. Inspirational, full of self-deprecating humour and frank emotion, Michael reveals his battle with ever-encroaching physical degeneration and how, together with the support of family and friends, outright victory for the disease is anything but assured. This book gives the ammunition to fight back and the courage to confront head on any terminal disease, and is a must-read for those facing such a diagnosis, their families and friends.' – **Jean Waters,** trustee of the Motor Neurone Disease Association (and a sufferer from MND)

To my family,
through whom and from whom I have
experienced God's love

Foreword

Michael's book is a true story. It is not triumphalistic as so many are; it is a true story of his encounter with a terminal illness. It is a true story of his refusal to give up. It is an encounter of one who remains a vicar of three parishes despite his deteriorating health. It is a truthful encounter of a willingness to engage with what the Almighty is doing and saying amongst his personal tragedy. I read this in Baghdad where I work. I love reading, I love studying books, but for the first time in years I was driven to tears by this book. Tears because of Michael's suffering, tears because of his refusal to give up and tears because I had the realization that I also have a neurological illness with many of the symptoms, though not as severe as Michael endures.

Among his writing there is the immense care and appreciation for the one who cares for him, his wife Jane. A care and love that it is also difficult to mention without knowing the pain caused to one's loved ones through chronic illness. The questions that Michael asks are questions that all people of faith ask when going through the 'valley of the shadow of death'. This book is honest; it is truthful, but it is not without hope. It is a hope that despite all odds you can keep going; despite the difficulties and questions our God will not leave us and, despite the feelings of many, even those who have lost much can give much.

Reading this book is entering into the reality of both a God and his people who suffer. It does not provide all the answers, but it does ask many of the questions. Questions I myself ask here in Baghdad. As I write, I hear the shooting and the rockets flying, but it is the questions that Michael asks that are the true questions of life and death. 'Even though I walk through the valley of the shadow of death, I will fear no evil because thy rod and staff comfort me'. Yesterday as I took the service in the US Embassy chapel, the rockets came in. The congregation took to the ground, continuing to sing the hymn 'No never alone'. Michael's book, *My Donkeybody,* tells a true story that despite all odds we are never alone.

Andrew White
Baghdad, June 2008

Acknowledgments

The journey which this little book is to describe was very agreeable and fortunate for me. After an uncouth beginning, I had the best of luck to the end. But we are all travellers in what John Bunyan calls the wilderness of this world – all, too, travellers with a donkey: and the best that we find in our travels is an honest friend. He is a fortunate voyager who finds many. We travel, indeed, to find them. They are the end and the reward of life. They keep us worthy of ourselves; and when we are alone, we are only nearer to the absent.

Every book is, in an intimate sense, a circular letter to the friends of him who writes it. They alone take his meaning; they find private messages, assurances of love, and expressions of gratitude, dropped for them in every corner. The public is but a generous patron who defrays the postage...

(Robert Louis Stevenson, *Travels with a Donkey in the Cevennes,* C. Kegan Paul, 1879: dedication)

There are many friends who in one way or another have contributed to the writing of this book. First and foremost are my wife and best friend, Jane, and my amazing children, Rachel, Paul and his wife Penny, Stephen and Bryan, whom I love more than I can say. Secondly, there are those who have travelled with me on my journey, some of whom are mentioned in the pages that follow, most of whom are not. In particular, thank you, Louise, for originally inspiring me with your honesty in 2006 and encouraging me since. Thirdly, I want to thank the remarkable church family in Stanford in the Vale, of which I'm privileged to be a part. Fourthly, I want to acknowledge those who have had and are having a far harder experience of terminal illness than mine has been so far. I hope you will forgive me if it feels that I have made light of your agony in any way. It's true, as the old slaves' spiritual says, 'Nobody knows de trouble I've seen...' I must also say a deep thank you to Andrew White who found time in his life of faith and danger to write a foreword for me. I was overwhelmed by his generous spirit. Finally, thank you to Tony Collins, who has been such an affirming editor for a rookie author.

Ad maiorem Dei gloriam
(For the greater glory of God)

Introduction

'You must tell your story'

I have an aversion to people making capital out of their own, or others', 'misfortunes'. It seems to me somehow cheapening. It smacks of sensational journalism – the sort that makes a story out of domestic tragedy in order to sell its paper or programme. I once knew a baby who was severely scalded when his mother had a seizure. I remember the story appearing nationally, after the ambulance message (as he was rushed to hospital) had been intercepted by someone who made it his business to listen to the emergency frequencies. It wasn't national news; it was simply an ordinary family in distress, who wanted to be left to cope in peace.

My story is not news either. It is what is happening in thousands of homes in Britain, and really no different from millions in the world. I'm no more special than the thousands with degenerative diseases, nor more interesting than any one of the millions facing premature death. Not more; not less. On government databases merely a statistic, but ultimately a unique individual. These are not, after all, the days of kings and queens, popes and bishops, the great and the good. The Spirit is poured out on the whole gamut of humankind. Tragedies befall salesmen. Today, celebrity is thrust upon the ordinary.

However, this is not about celebrity; nor is it a tragedy. It's more the passing on of a whisper. In *The Nun's Priest's Tale* by Chaucer, retelling the classical legend, King Midas tries to conceal his donkey-like ears under his hat, but the reeds where he swims in the river whisper his secret on the breeze: 'Midas has asses' ears.' Mine is not exactly a secret, because those who know me cannot help but notice that my body is less and less doing what I want. I have a stubborn ass of a body with shuffling legs and a braying laugh.

Of course, I am not alone. The world is full of people struggling to carry on in spite of the pains and protests of the physical body which carries them. The name of my particular condition, which I share with about 5,000 other people in the UK, is motor neurone disease (Amyotrophic Lateral Sclerosis elsewhere, and often Lou Gehrig's in the USA); but there are plenty more – common and uncommon – names for what is in the end a universal condition, mortality: multiple sclerosis, muscular dystrophy, Parkinson's disease, Huntington's chorea, cystic fibrosis, Alzheimer's disease, cancer, depression...

I think it is for the sake of such people, and for those who grieve and care for them, that different individuals have encouraged me to tell my story: to whisper it on the breeze. Certainly it is for you, fellow travellers, that I am writing. I must admit that it is also for myself, as I enjoy putting my thoughts on paper, and doubtless the whole process has therapeutic elements in it. In coming out, I am aware that I have seen very little yet. Though I have totally lost my independence, I am able to sit up and type this. I can even – with severe limitations and a great deal of help – carry on my job. I am a vicar: that is, I look after three churches between Oxford and Swindon in mid-England. I suppose there's an unspoken expectation on the part of many that my job includes justifying the ways of God (if there is one) to men. However, my present aim is not to square that circle, because I cannot do it. Yet, as I tell my story, there may emerge some shafts of light. Let's hope so; otherwise you're in for a dismal read. Well, here goes.

Chapter One

Cracks Begin to Appear

Loch Moidart, Western Scotland, July 2001. Castle Tioram stands on a tidal island near the southern shore. It's a romantic ruin, but its history is closely tied up with the tragic events of the Jacobite uprising and the ruthless Highland Clearances. From it the Silver Walk, a path marked as 'dangerous', runs east along the rocky shore, rising and falling on the wooded cliff, revealing views down to the beach and across the loch.

We're on holiday – four weeks away from work – the first such prolonged break in fifteen years. Jane, my wife, and I are on our own, staying in a gatekeeper's cottage on the Kinlochmoidart estate. Swallows nest in the eaves. It is a full-bloomed summer. Today we are visiting the castle built by the Macdonalds of Clan Ranald and have identified this lochside walk for after lunch. We set out through the evergreen laurels.

We come to a point where the path narrows round a blind bend. It's not that far above the loch, but my nerve suddenly fails. I find myself frozen to the spot, and cling to Jane. I cannot go on. This has never happened to me before. Heights have held no terrors for me in the past. I enjoyed scaling the Avon Gorge when a boy, climbing Mount Kenya in my teens and nipping up and down church towers in my job. This is irrational – cowardly – unmanly. However, I cannot argue myself round that corner, and after several long minutes, as it feels, we turn back. Jane does not seem desperately disillusioned by this onset of wimpishness, but I feel a failure. It has been a long haul, mark you, and the last few months at work have been particularly stressful. So perhaps I am just tired.

That holiday did not succeed in putting me right back on my feet. My confidence had been undermined. Although to all outward appearances nothing was different, as with subterranean tunnelling, the building was not quite as safe. And then there was the voice... Nevertheless, it was a glorious ten days in the most beautiful corner of Scotland: a great northern diver in a high loch, red deer in the wild, walks up hills and over to St Finnan's island, orchids and meadowsweet in profusion, and endlessly changing views. Our last day coincided with a wedding on the estate, and we went to sleep watching a firework display in the glen.

Our next staging post was a large house overlooking the Clyde, Kilcreggan, where we had booked in for a few nights' bed and breakfast. Just round the corner is Faslane naval base, where Britain's Trident submarines have their home. It is an area of the highest security and, one senses, intense surveillance. But the house is a haven of calm and hospitality. A turreted Victorian pile typical of Scotland, it once played host to missionaries recovering from their exertions in the colonies. Since then it has fallen on hard times, and now a couple, Peter and Nancy

Stanway, are trying to revive its fortunes and establish a faith community there. Peter spends much of his time in Glasgow's East End working with a church community project.

So we found ourselves in not quite your run-of-the-mill B and B. Yet it was not the wide, sweeping oak staircase as we entered, nor the ceiling-high bay window in our room with its panoramic view over the river that impressed me, but the cream-coloured slip of paper on my side of the bed. After the welcome, it read: '"For I know the plans I have for you," declares the LORD, "plans to prosper you and not to harm you, plans to give you hope and a future." Jeremiah 29:11'.

'That's nice,' I thought, and kept it as a bookmark. Little did I realize then what significance this would assume for me later. On our wedding anniversary we visited Helensburgh and had a celebratory tea. In one shop we found a bone china mug decorated with many of the flowers we'd seen in the hills around Loch Moidart, and bought it as a souvenir.

We needed those few days being looked after, as the next fortnight was spent running and catering for a camp of more than a hundred young people in the Lake District, at the end of which, drained, I noted, 'I feel wobbly and panicky.' It was not quite how I had anticipated finishing my restorative break.

I returned home to take a big funeral for a much-loved neighbour who had endured many years of gradually degenerating health, looked after by her distinguished and faithful husband. Letty Hamilton-Baillie had never given up. With irrepressible and forthright humour, she was the epitome of hospitality. The pancake party they threw every Shrove Tuesday was a village legend. Even though wheelchair-bound for years, she would not be confined. With Lottie, her pekinese, ensconced in the basket at the front, she would set off fearlessly (recklessly in the opinion of some) for a 'walk' down the track out of the village, occasionally overturning and having to wait for rescue until someone would come past and raise help. She died at home. Her grave is just over our garden wall. Jock, her husband, died a year later and is buried next to her.

Chapter Two

The Voice

The hoarseness would not go away. It was not a sore throat. My voice simply would not sound normal. And on one occasion I lost a word in the bath. I was in mid-sentence to Jane and, out of the blue, I could not get my tongue round some word or other. This had been before the summer and, since it had shown no sign of improving by September, when the pace of work picks up, I went to my GP, Sarah Shackleton. She must have examined the obvious things and, I suppose, made a shortlist of possibilities. She did not dismiss it lightly, but referred me to the ear, nose and throat (ENT) consultant, who held a clinic at the practice. And so began a year-long series of appointments: a winding road with an unknown destination.

Now in my job, my voice is an important part of my equipment. So for it to lose its tone – to become flat and slightly slurred – was an inconvenience, to say the least. People in the churches where I worked were too polite to mention it (at least to my face), and I carried on as normal, with the usual round of meetings, services and visits. However, an outspoken friend and a concerned brother bluntly commented on what was happening to me.

One night, the telephone rang. It was Rob, my friend from university days. I took it in the bedroom, with the usual greeting: 'Rob, how nice to hear you!'

'Mike, you're drunk.' Whether he was hoping it might be so, or simply an experienced diagnosis, it was actually untrue, and I told him so. I don't remember what explanation I gave him, but no doubt it was unsatisfactory. I could not explain it to myself.

A short time after this I received a call from my eldest brother, Gordon, in the course of which he said, 'Michael, you sound as though you've had a stroke...' We all knew what that sounded like, since my father had suffered from strokes for some years before he died. Were my words really coming out like that, slurred and sideways? Reality began to check in. And of course, I did not want to hear that I might have a problem of that magnitude.

In November a former parishioner dared to tell me about telephones that were able to amplify your voice, which would 'relieve the strain', and then, one Friday evening at the village youth club, some local teenagers plucked up courage to suggest to me that I was getting too fond of my drink (actually, more like ''Ere, you're f***ing pissed, ain't you, Vicar?'). I am sure my reassurances did not wash with them, and the 'fact' that the vicar had taken to drink circulated round the parish. It was of a different order from the very audible comment made many years earlier by an old villager witnessing the new vicar as I finished the unconsumed communion wine: ''E do like his drink, that vicar, don't he?' Village rumours with an edge of the scandalous or malicious have an energy of their own. There is nothing you can do to dispel them. So I did not bother to try.

Chapter Three

Testing, Testing...

Meanwhile, I was being investigated. The ear, nose and throat specialist looked down the relevant orifices and found nothing abnormal. Which was, in one way, good news, but in another was the opposite, as my doctor at once made an appointment with the neurology department at the old Radcliffe Infirmary in Oxford, where Jane had worked as a physiotherapist before we were married and where my father had been an in-patient after his strokes. It was not the first time I had been back to the hospital corridors after his death, as my job had taken me there on visits to people from the parish after cancer and eye operations. (As well as the brain, the same site dealt with eyes, ears, noses and throats.) It was, however, my first experience of being a patient, and neurology sounds a bit alarming. My appointment came through quickly. The registrar set me going on a succession of tests and scans.

The first line of enquiry was to examine my muscles and nerve conduction, for which, via pads or needles, I was wired up to a computer. The doctor would carefully choose the points, fix or insert the electrodes, switch on the machine and watch. From time to time he would ask me to move the relevant limb, or relax. In some tests he'd warn me to expect a minor shock, and I'd watch my fingers or foot twitch. It felt a bit like what they used to do to frogs' legs in biology lessons to make them twitch, only it was a full-sized me. On one of the pincushion sessions, the sort in which needles were stuck into various parts of my body to measure the speed with which the messages travelled through my nervous system, something went wrong. The results did not come out properly. I seem to remember that the computer was suffering from interference. So I had to return to have more needles inserted in my tongue: painlessly, I was relieved to discover. Nothing much seemed to be showing up, but it was all being recorded. I was alive and kicking, at least. Then came the MRI scan, with the customary stories about the tunnel inches above your eyes and the ensuing claustrophobic panic.

The day before my scan, we visited our good friends John and Mary. We had met them in the year we were married, when my first teaching job was in the town where John himself was vicar. Mary was an orthoptist at the same hospital where Jane was then working as a physio. It was a miracle that John was alive, since he had been struck down with a brain tumour four years previously, and there was little expectation that he would survive. However, he was rushed into the Infirmary, operated on, prayed for intensively and was and is very much and cheerfully alive. As a seasoned campaigner, he reassured me about MRIs. 'The thing is, there's nowhere God is not.

So I would say, "Jesus, come with me," and he did, and we'd spend the time together.' It was true. The radiologists carefully ensure that you have no metal objects on you or in you to fall foul of the massive magnetic forces in which you lie. But they don't ask you to leave God in the little locker in the anteroom, along with your watch, your wallet and your pen.

In the event, neither lying in that giant magnet nor later in the radiologists' equivalent of a bacon-slicer, the CT scanner, proved alarming, and the outcome of both was negative – or positive, depending on your outlook. In other words, no physical abnormalities showed up. My brain was there and intact. So they looked down my throat again, this time at the Infirmary. For once, the cracks in the National Health Service were exposed. Of the three consultants on clinic, one was ill, one was called to an emergency on the wards and one was left to cope. The waiting-room was packed and, in spite of the staff's best efforts, some patients lost it. Then came a Dickensian diversion. Two men in what can best be described as grey-blue boilersuits entered with an inoffensive-looking individual manacled between them. Jumping all the very long queues, they were ushered directly through to a consulting room. The frisson caused by the passage of this (clearly) dangerous criminal was soon enough absorbed by the heat and the renewed mutterings of discontent. In fact, as we later learned, he was probably no more than an unwell inmate of the demeaning Campsfield Immigration Detention

Centre. Such inmates, though far from dangerous, tended to be treated like high-security criminals.

For me, however, this examination revealed nothing new. Thus, in the spring of 2002 the doctors were keeping an open mind. It might be any one of a number of possibilities, including just a one-off freak condition, but there was no clear diagnosis. I would return in six months for another check-up.

Work and normal life carried on unabated, whilst I took some steps to alleviate the load of public speaking which is the staple fare of a vicar's job. The summer came and went, with another youth camp in the Lakes and a family holiday in North Wales with walks in the hills, including an ascent of the Snowdon Ranger path from Nantgwynant up to the summit.

Chapter Four

Among the Unsung

'This is a bit embarrassing. I've never done anything like this before in my life, but your brother mentioned that you were also living in this area and suggested we might like to meet up...' Thus I started a letter to a physiotherapy student at the London Hospital in Whitechapel in 1971.

I was living in Hoxton Square, Shoreditch, years before it had become fashionable. It was then full of warehouses and small factory units, with the exception of one relic of the past, The Vicarage, where a number of medical students and assorted graduates lodged. On leaving university, I had begun my first job, in Bedford Square, as an editorial assistant in a small religious publishing house. London life was endlessly stimulating. In spite of somewhat regimented and claustrophobic digs, I loved it. I loved Shoreditch, with its amazingly welcoming people, who lived in monstrous tower-block flats, and I loved the West End, with its mixture of gentility and sleaze, where I was part of the rivers of office-workers flowing in and out like a morning and evening tide.

Having posted the letter, I waited for a reply, which came, as I remember, by telephone. 'There's a girl on the phone for you, Michael,' I was told one evening at tea, with ill-disguised curiosity. So began a lifelong friendship.

It is high time to introduce Jane, my partner and wife, in more depth, as this book is as much about her as about me.

It's late autumn. I am waiting at the road entrance to Waterloo underground station, which is where we had agreed to meet, to have a meal before a concert at the Festival Hall. I suppose there were others being disgorged from below, but I see only one. She is not tall, nor dressed to kill. In fact she is wearing a yellowish raincoat. She has naturally curly brown hair and very nice ankles. As she comes closer, I like what I see: she has an open face, neatly defined eyebrows, full lips, small nose and deep honest eyes. What she sees in me I don't stop to think.

Whatever it was, it was not love at first sight, nor was it a whirlwind romance. However, when I moved out to share a rented house in Ealing with a college friend, and when I changed jobs early in 1973 to become a hospital porter on the way to teaching, it became clear that Jane was more important to me than other friends. My black split-screen Morris Minor grew accustomed to the evening journey along Western Avenue, along the Marylebone Road, through Euston and Dalston to Kenninghall Road, Clapton, and back before midnight. Films, meals, concerts, theatre in Regent's Park ... and then, as the story goes, 'he came to himself and said': 'How many weeks do you have left?' Jane's course was nearing its end. Her finals were in June; and then she would move back to stay with her parents in Brentwood, Essex, where her father taught. It was 'make your mind up time'. The evening before her final examination, the viva, Jane invited me to a last meal in her flat. I parked the old car in the road outside, and rang the bell. Up the three flights of stairs, to the flat Jane shared with two other physio students. One was engaged; the other had a boyfriend, who was a medical student. I assumed they were in their rooms. One of them certainly was. Carol, vivacious and glamorous, was playing the orchestral version of *Pictures at an Exhibition* by Mussorgsky – which needs to be loud, and was. For me it will always be connected with that flat and that evening. I don't remember what we talked about. Jane had things to think about before the night was out, such as her final revision. So did I. Before leaving I had to take the plunge.

'I've a question to ask ... Will you marry me?'

Silence. A long wait.

'Well, the answer's not no.'

Ever since, it has been held against me (by all but Jane) as an example of crass insensitivity that it was then that I asked her to marry me – the night before the most important exam in her life. The consequence could have been disastrous.

In the event it was not, though more as a result of her assiduousness than of my timing. She emerged with a distinction – because she was smiling, according to her. For me, the outcome was less satisfactory, at least temporarily, as she had not said yes, and I was left hanging. There was a certain poetic justice about it. And maybe, in retrospect, the magnitude of what she would have been undertaking should have given pause for thought. However, a few weeks later, when she was on holiday in her parents' home in the Isle of Wight, I was catering at a youth camp along the coast at Bembridge. In an afternoon break we met and walked along the cliff path, which twisted in and out of the gorse and windswept bushes. She had something to tell me: 'I think I know what the answer is now.' And that was all. I was too tired to handle momentous news, and anyhow in a couple of days I would spend a night at the house in Seaview. So we left it on hold and enjoyed the sun and the sea.

Two days later, after supper, we walked down Gully Road to the beach. It was getting dark. The tide was out, so it was possible to walk out onto the sand. Whether the moon was out or not, I don't know. We strolled along the beach towards Priory Bay, the woods tumbling right down to the sea's edge, and stopped before the rocks began to stretch out, defining the bays. The lights of Southsea flickered across the Solent.

'The answer is yes.'

It was pitch dark when we retraced our steps up the steep hill, with houses on one side and trees overhanging on the other. It must have been apparent to Jane's parents that the question had been asked and answered, but with great restraint they didn't pry. It was only after a return journey to my family home in Oxfordshire and the purchase of a ring that I formally asked Dennis Tarrant for permission to marry his daughter. He also said yes.

Chapter Five

For Better, for Worse

So began eleven months of engagement, while I trained for teaching in Nottingham and Jane began work as a physiotherapist in the Radcliffe Infirmary. I wouldn't describe those months as stormy, but from time to time the sea had threatening white horses. Glandular fever disrupted my teaching practice, and there was the possibility of postponing qualification. I disagreed stubbornly with the rector of the church where we planned to be married, about his part in the service. It might be *his* church, but it was *our* wedding, I reasoned. His perspective was a bit different. Jane endured some fairly miserable weekend visits to Nottingham. During the course of one of them I had reached the point of giving everything up. In this instance music was the food of love, as we went to a concert of Mozart and Schubert given by the London Symphony Orchestra in the City Hall. The cycle of introversion was broken during those two hours, and life seemed good again. Jane was relieved!

A few months later, on 20 July, when I had just completed my training as a teacher, we were married. My father married us, the rector blessed us and Jane's godfather preached. Coincidentally, Meredith Dewey had also been dean of my college, so he knew us both well. 'There is always a vein of melancholy in a marriage,' he said. 'For those who listen to your irrevocable vows of generosity and fidelity, laughter and tears pulse together like stars in a polar sky, indelibly bright but unattainably remote. Laughter because we rejoice in your happiness. Tears because your love reminds us of our lost primal innocence – described by Milton's last lines to his epic: "They, hand in hand, with wandering steps and slow, through Eden took their solitary way." The world may crash around you, the times are unsettled. But you have each other. Every sorrow shared is half endured. Every joy enjoyed together a special felicity, every laugh a double laugh.' He talked about the spring and the autumn of love. 'For you this day is spring, not autumn. You now have the unexampled felicity of getting to know one another through the ups and downs of life, in prosperity and adversity. To know one other person through and through – that is how St Paul describes heaven in his deathless hymn to charity: "Then shall I know, even as I am known."' He was a poet, as well as a priest; maybe he was a prophet as well.

The following September, I began teaching at Buntingford, in the north of Hertfordshire, and Jane found a new job in Hertford Hospital. The spring of our love began in a condemned council house in Bishop's Stortford with one cold water tap and an outside toilet, shared with scores of snails. It was damp and draughty, but it was our first home. We were happy. With both of us having to travel to work, we wanted to buy a house where one of us worked, when we could afford it. In the end we found a Victorian labourer's cottage on the edge of Buntingford, which had been put on the map by a large Sainsbury's depot with its accompanying housing estate, from where many of our pupils came. A couple of them hit the tabloids by eloping to Gretna Green. The staff at school weren't too surprised. Two years later, Jane went as an in-patient to the hospital where she worked. Rachel was born in May, and Jane became a full-time mother. My career took me to two further schools. Eight years, three houses and three children later, we were in Oxford, I was once more considering a career change, and Jane was facing yet another call on her tolerance.

Having married a teacher with good prospects and with her own career stretching ahead of her, she had suspended her vocation and exchanged it for that of running a home. When my mother was killed in a road accident in 1980, Jane's family was increased by the addition of my kindly but undomesticated father, who came to live with us. I had reached a crossroads in my teaching. I began to apply for deputies' jobs and headships and to go for interviews.

At the same time, however, I was being nudged in a different direction, and after the customary lengthy selection procedure I ended up being accepted for training to become a 'reverend' in the Church of England. So now Jane would be asked to manage a household of seven on a student grant for two years and, ultimately, to become that modern anomaly, the vicar's wife. In due course it would mean leaving a beautiful home by the Oxford Canal and a circle of close friends, and in the event moving away to Hazel Grove in the borough of Stockport, on the edge of Manchester. All this she faced with equanimity. But I had something more in store for her.

On the day of the move, Jane took the younger children to the primary school, about fifteen minutes' walk away, while I awaited the arrival of the removal men. She returned to find the vans parked outside with the men still sitting in them. Why no action? We had moved often enough to know that removers do not waste much time. Entering by the side gate, she came in through the kitchen door and was confronted by my father and one of my fellow students, who happened to be a doctor, and my recumbent confused self on the floor. No one had been around when I had blacked out by the back door, and I had complete memory loss. One thing was clear: moving was out of the question, at least for a week, and driving would be unwise. Accident and Emergency at the John Radcliffe Hospital came up with no conclusive diagnosis, and so I was referred to the Manchester Royal Infirmary for investigations after we had moved.

In due course it was reckoned to have been an epileptic fit, which was acutely confirmed when I had another *grand mal* seizure on packing up at the end of a shared holiday in the Brecon Beacons. This time Jane was there to witness her unconscious husband gnashing and thrashing on the ground. There was no doubt I had developed epilepsy. I was put on one of the standard drugs, but that did not prevent me having three more major fits, one when I was standing behind the altar-table about to celebrate communion on Good Friday in my new parish in rural Oxfordshire. I shall not forget the hushed voices of concern echoing in the medieval church as I came round, and the reassuring sight of Jane leaning over, telling me what had happened, before I was taken to the ambulance. A change of medication succeeded in controlling the fits, and I have had none since. Nevertheless, for Jane, it became like living with an unpredictable time-bomb.

Not that she betrayed her anxiety or fear. In fact I – and she – discovered strengths in her which had not been obvious before. To take a quite mundane example: after fits, of course, I was not allowed to drive. Our 'car' was a Volkswagen camper van. On one occasion, we had a camping holiday in France planned, when suddenly I could not drive. So Jane did, also shouldering an unequal share of parenting until I regained my licence. I should have felt guilty. Perhaps I did, but she kept on keeping on. Admiration was added to my affection. It was not all adversity, however. These were dark moments in an increasingly close and happy relationship. After the rain, the blackbird sings.

I suppose we are now in the autumn of our love, with the winds blowing the leaves off the trees. However, Jane is still with me.

One evening during the weeks following Hurricane Katrina in 2005, when television pictures of that devastation in New Orleans had first invaded our living room, I sat at the table after one supper watching Jane clearing up in the kitchen. It used to be a shared activity, from preparing to eating and to washing. Now all I could contribute was to eat and sit and watch, and I realized how disproportionate Jane's part of the marriage contract had become. It was so unfair. At that moment I hated it: the frustration, the impotence and, above all, Jane's undeserved burden. So I wrote:

Storm Service

Through the open door,
bending over used plates, piled pots and stained cutlery,
I see my wife, skivvying.
The fresh bloom battered by unlooked-for whirlwinds.
Is this service, or is it slavery?
It wasn't in the brochures–
with their pictures of sun-basking villas,
pristine palaces for the moderately well-off.
'Yes, it was. Look, here, sir. In the small print:
No guarantee. *' 'Better, or worse.'*
Tropical paradise, or hurricane hell.

But this is a force ten, rising;
and the levees have never been tested like this before.
You assure me that roots are made stronger;
rubbish is stripped away;
goodness rises from ruins.
Maybe that's true.
But now I see the wind-bowed palm in the colour-extinguishing fury,
a repeating loop of incremental intensity–
crying, 'How long?'

Chapter Six

What's Wrong?

After the summer, my six months were up – and it was back to the Infirmary for more appointments and more tests. These were annoying not because they were painful, but because they invariably fell on my day off. It seemed a waste. Some wits, imagining themselves to be original, say vicars work one day a week. Not where I come from! Certainly they have to work on Sundays; but the days of gentlemen clergy who mooch in their studies and potter in their gardens are long gone. The most popular day off seems to be Monday, but mine has always been Tuesday, and Tuesday is the day of the Neurology outpatient clinics. So we would set off for Oxford, round the infamous ring road (which must be the most-mentioned A road on traffic reports: 'The A34 at Peartree Roundabout'), down the Woodstock Road and hunt down that rarity, the two-hour parking space in central Oxford. We usually struck gold in Observatory Street, from where it was a short walk to the hospital. Then came the waiting, followed by the appointment. Once that was finished and the journey home completed, a substantial part of the day had been used up.

Although the junior doctors refrained from hazarding guesses, I gathered that they were doing their detective work and working on some hypothesis. I was also making my own guesses. On the penultimate appointment of 2002, I saw a senior house officer and decided to try them out. I gave him a short list of three: 'Might it be Parkinson's, or MS, or some sort of stroke?' He was cautious, but we came away with the impression that it probably was not one of them, but perhaps something more unusual.

'Revd Wenham, would you like to sit down?' What is it about the formality of 'Reverend' that alerts me to ominous news ahead?

(What a ridiculous anachronism that word is, anyway! Was it invented by clergy to disguise the truth, or to express a devout wish? 'To be revered' – give us a break! Under these clothes and titles, I'm no different from the rest of humanity, from Edgar, alias poor Tom, in *King Lear*: 'unaccommodated man is no more but such a poor, bare, forked animal as thou art.'[1] As for 'Venerable' and 'Very' and 'Right' Reverends, they seem to me the height of pompous 'lendings'. I regularly receive letters starting, 'Dear the Reverend Mr Michael Wenham.' What's wrong with plain Mr? It seems to me that to parade titles and qualifications is a sign of insecurity.)

This time, we have finally reached the session with the main man: the consultant himself. I have sat down. 'My colleagues have done all the tests and, having examined them and seen you today, I'm afraid I agree with their conclusion: that they all point to your having a motor neurone disorder.' Michael Donaghy was direct in confirming my worst-case scenario to Jane and me. This was the big one. I knew about David Niven and Peter Cook. And it was not so long ago that Diane Pretty had been on the television news, pleading through her husband to be put out of her misery: her life which was no life. She had died in May. I knew, without needing to ask, that there was no cure. It was a death sentence.

My mind did not go blank. I don't think I went into denial, more into a curious detachment. This was undoubtedly happening to me. I – yes, I, Michael Wenham – had MND, the dreaded degenerative condition. But the only question I could think to ask was, 'How long do you think I've got?' To which I received the predictable, but honest, answer that it was impossible to say. It affected individuals differently, but I seemed to have a more slowly developing type. (Do I mentally cling like a drowning man to the remarkable Professor Stephen Hawking?) There was no surfacing emotion, no protesting that it must be a mistake. Just a matter-of-fact feeling, 'Well, that's it, then.' Presumably Dr Donaghy made the appropriate concluding remarks about writing to the GP and making the next appointment. I honestly do not remember. But I intended no irony when I thanked him. And so we stepped out into the crowded clinic waiting room.

Things there looked no different from when I had been called into the consulting room. Receptionists and nurses were carrying on as normal; patients and carers were sitting, waiting, reading and watching the world go by; children were getting fractious. Yet the world – my world – was different. It had changed beyond recognition; perhaps beyond redemption. 'God's in his heaven and all's well with the world.' But not with mine. All I knew now was what was wrong with me. Strangely, although the news was profoundly shocking, it did not seem to have power over us. Psychologists might well identify this as the numb stage of grief, or simply as denial. Maybe they would be right. But at no stage was I inclined to deny either the accuracy of the diagnosis or the reality of the condition. When you are inside it, you are not in a position to say, 'This is not happening to me.' You feel it in your muscles. You see it in other people's eyes.

I was aware, however, of the power of the curse. By that I do not mean some malign spell deliberately cast over some unfortunate person, but simply the power for the worse we allow words to exercise over our lives. Whether it is a child being told by a teacher, 'You'll never be any good,' or an adult being told by a doctor, 'It's cancer,' FAILURE and DEATH are printed like ineradicable subtitles across every frame of our life from then on. Each new day, unfolding before us, has the curse stamped across it. Failure ... Failure ... Failure..., or Death ... Death ... Death ... And of course we believe it, because the teacher said so, the doctor said so, the authority said so. The truth is that it may well be that we will never make it as a premiership footballer, or that our cancer will be terminal, but yet it is *not* inevitable. The curse can so easily snuff out hope.

Somehow, my diagnosis did not have that effect on me. Maybe it was because facing death and dying is such an integral part of my job. Every burial and cremation I take, I say: 'The days of man are but as grass. He flourishes like the flower of the field. The wind blows over it and it is gone, and its place will be remembered no more.' From premature babies to centenarians; from close family to complete strangers; heroes to wastrels; I have buried them all. I know that life is essentially fragile. The issue is what we do with whatever interim we have. Or maybe it was to do with the prayers of our friends, who were aware of my progress through the clinics. I have no doubt that prayer was to play a significant part in the battle between hope and despair that would loom in the days ahead.

There was not much to say as we walked through the corridors and out of the hospital's front doors into the courtyard, with its central fountain playing in the October morning sunshine. We decided against calling on my brother David, who worked in that part of Oxford. Instead we went into the centre to buy a pullover from the Edinburgh Woollen Mill, and found there a mug identical to the one we'd bought on our Scottish holiday and since broken. We sauntered back down jostling Cornmarket, the familiar shopping street, and tree-lined St Giles. The bicycles and cars passed on the Woodstock Road. A small queue waited at the bus stop. Were any of them, I wondered, nursing an acute diagnosis – as acute as mine? We headed back to the car, past the former Clarendon Observatory, and drove home to the Vicarage, where we clung to each other. Twenty-nine years before, on a clear August evening, we had stood beneath the huge walnut tree in the grounds of my parents' old vicarage, in Lowford, the mother village of 'Larkrise' to the east of Oxford, and clung to each other in our first passionate embrace. It was – is – still a vivid memory. Was it to end so soon? Was this the beginning of the final whimper?

Note

[1] William Shakespeare, *King Lear,* 3.4.109 (Arden edition, 1964).

Chapter Seven

Breaking Bad News

We decided that our children had to be the first to know, and that we should tell them directly, if possible, not by telephone. With the exception of Paul, who was married and living in Manchester, it was possible, as they all happened to come or be at home during that week. We did not over-dramatize the news, but I was unable to keep the gravity of the diagnosis out of my voice. Indeed, for a long time I simply found it hard to articulate the very words 'motor neurone disease'. I could not pretend that it did not affect me. As for Rachel, Stephen and Bryan – well, there is not much to say when your father announces such news. Sometimes, perhaps especially within close families, words are unnecessary, even get in the way. That evening there was eloquent silence – and I guess some tears.

We then informed our wider family and my boss, Dominic Walker, the Bishop of Reading. He emailed back, expressing his sympathy, of course, but more significantly saying that ministry could be strengthened by weakness. This was the first of two seemingly similar, but profoundly different responses I learned to identify over the coming days and months. I would call one 'simple sympathy' and the other 'faith-informed sympathy'. The former is negative in effect, albeit unintentionally, and the latter is positive in effect and in intention. A couple walk down the drive and ring the bell. 'We are so sorry to hear your dreadful news, Michael. Do tell us if we can ever help at all.' Somehow, as they retreat, it feels as though they have begun the countdown to the inevitable, like latter-day *tricoteuses.* Or a well-meaning carer in the local nursing home greets me, unusually, on one of my regular visits. She is sorry to hear my news. Her father died of motor neurone disease six months before. It is, she says, like a coma in reverse; your mind is fully alert, while your body is utterly inert. Though this shows a greater degree of understanding than average, which is welcome, strangely it is not the sort of news one needs to hear early on. It goes with the downturned mouth and the large 'You-poor-poor-man' eyes. Usually it is kindly meant. Yet if you are not ready for it, it saps hope and even life out of you, drop by drop.

After our family, it was time to inform the church. It was the last Sunday in October. I decided not to make a drama out of it... So I put a short note about the consultant's diagnosis in the weekly news-sheet that was given to everyone as they came to the main service. It was a 'normal' service, following a set pattern. I don't remember what I preached about, but I wanted to end, I remember, with an extract from a letter I had recently received from Sarah Casson, a friend who was hoping to work in Congo. Her profession was translating the Bible.

The town of Goma, Congo, on the shores of Lake Kivu and the Rwandan border, has made international headlines twice in the past ten years. In 1994 thousands of Rwandan refugees streamed into it in the aftermath of the Rwandan genocide. In January of this year Goma found itself in the glare of the world's TV cameras again when Mount Nyiragongo, the flat-topped volcano which dominates the town, erupted, engulfing a third of the town in a molten sea.

Goma has a special significance for me. It's the only place in the Democratic Republic of Congo I have been able to visit so far ... there a year ago I first sensed the whisperings of a 'call', if you want to put it like that, to Congo... I was blown away by the warmth, generosity and determination of Congolese colleagues who persevered with work on their language in the face of the suffering and deprivation brought by war. I was captivated by the rhythms and harmonies of the exuberant Congolese singing. So when at the beginning of this year I was offered a place on a special plane being chartered to take people (and books!) to the dedication of the gospel of Luke in Chitembo, I jumped at the chance to join in the celebrations...

The climax to the celebration came as the provincial head of the churches pulled a brilliant blue copy of Luke out of the boxes carefully placed at the front of the church, and amid clapping and cheering waved it triumphantly above his head for everyone to see. Then a hush fell as Pastor Bitwonga, one of the translators, read the story of the Good Samaritan from the new translation for the first time. People have not had much to celebrate about in Goma in the past months. Here at last was something to dance about, good news in the language they understood best, about the life and hope that Jesus brings, which no disaster, however devastating, can take away.

(As I am writing this, on holiday in France, a delicate scarlet and black beetle has walked across me and is resting on the edge of my notebook. It has a minute black dot on each wing, and a tear-shaped black mark at the back with a single point of light in the middle. Even in nature, it seems, darkness and light, beauty and tears mingle together.)

There is something about being surrounded by people who care about you which has peculiar power when you are vulnerable. Add to that the profound conviction that you have heard the truth, and it is for you, and you have an explosive mixture. As a young member of our church read out that final sentence from Sarah's letter, the explosion was detonated inside me and I wept. Not polite discreet tears, but howling uncontrollable sobs, echoing round the church.

It was an unscripted 'make-or-break' moment for the church. It's not often that a vicar totally loses the plot so publicly – rather like a performer on stage freezing beneath the spotlights. The audience has no way of telling what's happened to him, or when it will end. Who could tell what was going on inside me at that moment? Was it a realization of devastating loss? Was it overwhelming self-pity? Was it despair? Whatever it was, it looked and sounded shocking. Far from being in control, as I was normally, there was nothing I could do to direct what happened next. I sat weeping in my seat in front of the ancient pulpit. My daughter and son who were in church that morning came over to be with me. It was, as a girl later told her mother, 'a strange service'. A young mother suddenly began to pray out loud, unscripted, which was not the custom, and certainly not hers. She talked in a clear voice, in words I was not fit to take in. As she spoke, calm seemed to settle over everyone, including eventually me. The service continued, ending with a great twenty-first-century hymn whose last verse includes the lines:

> *From life's first cry to final breath,*
> *Jesus commands my destiny.*[1]

Was it true? To what extent did I believe it? If you'd asked me then, I would have answered, 'I'm convinced it's true.' Do I still believe it – five years down the line?

Note

[1] Stuart Townsend, 'In Christ alone', © 2002 Kingsway Music.

Chapter Eight

Let Him Who Stands Take Care...

I shall return to that question later; but first, how has MND developed for me? Although there is a roughly predictable profile to the disorders that come under the generic title of motor neurone disease, my understanding is that people affected experience the symptoms quite individually. My subspecies was later confirmed to be primary lateral sclerosis, which can begin to show itself in the voice, and then in other parts. A characteristic symptom is a tightening of the muscles. When my consultant described this technically as 'spasticity', I remembered that old ignorant schoolboy insult for the unathletic: 'spaz'. So this is what it's really like.

I don't like to give the impression that my life at this point was a succession of hospital appointments and holidays. However, perhaps because I had time to notice it, or perhaps being a change of routine, on the next summer holiday things took an unwelcome turn. It was if, unseen, in some deep subterranean region, there was an imperceptible shifting of tectonic plates, from which tremors occasionally arose. They might have seemed isolated minor incidents, but now I knew them to be the outriders of something much bigger.

I am not sure whether at this stage I had even begun to connect what had happened two summers previously in Scotland with my MND. However, Spain changed that. Some good friends offered us their apartment overlooking the Mediterranean Sea near Calpe. It was a welcome and convenient break. Our youngest son, Bryan, had finished his A levels; his older brother, Stephen, was about to graduate at Bristol University. It was very bright and very hot. We would have our meals on the balcony, overlooking the bay dominated by the rump-backed rock of Calpe. We relaxed totally and did very little sight-seeing. We did, one day, drive down the coast and inland to les Fonts de l'Algar, a popular local beauty-spot of cascading waterfalls and deep pools, in a fertile area of orange and olive groves, between the coast and the rocky hills. Joining the crowds, we climbed the wooden walkways between the cafés and reached the stony path leading up to the higher reaches of the cascade. Onwards and upwards to one of the top pools, with Spanish families around us and some characters enjoying the cool of the water. At that point, I lost my footing on some rocks and found myself falling, entirely unable to recover my balance or check my fall – or to get up on my feet again. Blood poured from my leg, my side was grazed, wind was knocked out of me and for some time I could not speak. Solicitous

Spaniards surrounded us. Was it a heart attack? There was excited talk of the air ambulance. Stephen ran halfway down the track to the First Aid post and brought back with him two paramedics, complete with stretcher and rescue equipment. Strapped in, I was carted down to the hut, where iodine was liberally applied to bits of my anatomy. When the paramedics were satisfied I was in one piece, we were allowed to go on our way, I limping self-consciously with my war-paint and the rest of the family more subdued than when we'd set out.

I was a bit more cautious after that, but even so, on two more occasions on rocky places by the beaches I slipped and threatened a repeat performance. Because of my injuries I was not fit to drive our hire car, but with other drivers that did not limit us or do much to take the shine off the holiday. By the time we were flying back from Alicante to Bristol, however, the sombre realization had begun to settle: the damage among the neurones was spreading.

Back home, it would have not been obvious – at first. There was no one around when I misjudged the kerb and toppled off my bicycle. Or did emergency stops into our garage door. And no one knew of my general loss of confidence in my balance. I did not easily admit my increasing fragility. There were, however, plenty of people around when I tripped over a cable in church and went down, in the full rig-out of church robes, and had to be helped to my feet. And there were quite enough people, one evening in our local market town, when I collapsed at the edge of the pavement.

Our friends Anthony and Ruth were staying with us for a night in December. Anthony needed some antihistamines, so we drove together to Faringdon. While he was in the chemist, I was crossing back to the car. Suddenly, from the market-place, a car swept round the corner. I checked my progress, stepped back and found myself in the gutter.

My first instinct was to look round to see that none of my parishioners had witnessed my indignity. My next concern was how I was going to stand up again. At least two women passed on the pavement behind me. I don't blame them for not stopping and offering to help. At that point, I must have looked like a drunk who had just rolled out of the pub. All I could think of doing was to crawl across the pavement on my hands and knees and haul myself upright on the pub's drainpipe. No doubt other shoppers and shopkeepers who had a grandstand view from over the road thought the same as the two who had passed me.

There was one exception: the estate agent from the small office opposite came over as I inched my way to the vertical. 'Are you all right? Would you like a chair? Can I help?' There was something immensely touching about that one compassionate woman who risked a rude rebuff to her sympathy. It almost made the mishap worth it. I thanked her and told her that Anthony would be along shortly. I'd be all right waiting. She did not insist further, but indicated where she would be: within hailing distance if need be.

That night, under cover of darkness, I walked to church on my own, on the route I had used thousands of times. There is a junction of the ways, where the path from the church door slopes up to meet the path through the village. It is right in the middle of the churchyard, and is marked by a rather too tall Narnian lamp-post. That was as far as I reached before my nerve gave out. I knew – or thought I knew – that I would lose my balance on that slope and end up in another heap on the ground, unable to move. There was only one thing to do. Hang on to the lamp-post and wait for someone to rescue me. I could foresee myself having surreal conversations with dog-walkers or pub-goers. How do you ask people to give you, the vicar, a hand to get to the church door? And how do they do it? 'Just take my arm, Vicar...'?

Not surprisingly, people in the parish would not now be so fazed by the situation, and neither would I. But this was early days. So there I stand, clinging to the lamp-post, with its little circular disc threatening owners of incontinent dogs with £250 fines, in its circle of light in the blackness. The minutes tick by. No one comes. Nothing stirs in the graveyard. Actually it is not long – it just seems it – before I hear voices, and then the characteristic click of our back-garden gate opening and shutting. Rescue is on its way. Darkness hides the shame on my face, and perhaps my hoarseness disguises my fear. Pretence, however, is useless. MND is essentially public, in the same way as epilepsy. Unless you shut yourself away, at home or in a hermitage, it will out.

Chapter Nine

Helpers

First I took to using a stick – one of those fashionable mountain walking accessories bought in the Lake District; then, thanks indirectly to the excellent physiotherapist, Lesley Hoare, who had taken to visiting me, a sturdy metal NHS adjustable model, with its typical plastic ergonomic handle and its squat rubber bung ('ferrule' in the trade jargon). Before too long Lesley, anxious to prevent falling and injury, had introduced me to the invaluable Rollator, a cross between a zimmer frame and a shopping trolley. This is surprisingly manoeuvrable and sturdy and keeps one on one's feet as long as muscle-power in legs and hands allows. Its great virtue is to allow independent mobility to a basically unstable upright biped. Psychologically it makes you feel safe, but it can also make you dependent on it, so that you become reluctant to move without it. This is the dilemma a physio faces: preserving her patient's independence and mobility for as long as possible and at the same time minimizing risk from injury, which as the disease progresses becomes increasingly hard to deal with.

Lesley is lovely. First impressions: typical physio, white polo shirt with navy cardigan and matching navy trousers, white trainers, blond shoulder-length hair, energetic and five foot four. In my experience, however – and I'm married to one, remember – there are no stereotypical physiotherapists. Lesley proved no exception. She is a canny professional. Neurological cases are her speciality. I suspect she summed me up in more ways than the physical assessment she carried out on her first visit. She knew how much to push me to consider aids such as bath seats and grab rails. She told us as much as I wanted to hear and pointed me to the Motor Neurone Disease Association, the charity devoted to researching and relieving the illness. I think she placed me towards the awkward end of the spectrum of her clients. She works over a wide area of Oxfordshire; she drives out to see me regularly, and makes herself available by telephone in case of need. She consistently discusses what is happening and is utterly undogmatic. As her patient, you feel, you can go as fast or as slowly as you choose. The patient is respected – and the feelings are mutual.

It is thanks to two physiotherapists, one employed by the NHS and one who years ago committed herself to me in sickness and in health, Lesley and Jane, that I have not had more falls and am still more or less on my feet. On her visits, Lesley tells Jane what she is observing and what exercises may help and demonstrates them. They talk about muscle tone, dragging toes and the best way to avoid damage to joints. Jane does my stretching exercises, and she acts as my support when I walk distances.

I have had amazingly few falls since then, even though I am now as unstable as a flamingo in a wind tunnel. Not so long ago, one Saturday morning I sneezed and, despite grabbing a handrail, slithered to the floor. Descending proved easier than ascending, with legs which have minds of their own with frustratingly little intelligence and even less strength. So there I sat, meditating on life's small absurdities, until rescued by Jane and Peter, a friend of mine who used to play rugby. Some months before that, I had sampled something of what Lesley is trying to protect me from when out walking with Jess, our black-and-white blue-eyed mongrel dog. In a moment of inattention, she ran in front of me and I tripped over her extendable lead. I do not remember it happening. All I remember is sitting in our home, wondering what had been happening. I must have banged my head and had mild concussion. I was woozy for a couple of days, and distinctly did not enjoy the fact that I had lost an hour or so of my life. But it might have been much worse. It might have happened on the stairs, or on a busy road.

I began to identify people walking head-down and keeping close to the shopfronts. I recognized the concentration required for someone struggling to maintain their balance. Mostly, staying upright and walking or running is something we do instinctively, by reflex. When those instinctive reflexes are interfered with, you have to rely on other means: primarily sight and the conscious processing of data via your eyes. Imagine a satellite navigation system with a gremlin in it, so that you have to compensate by half a mile for all its instructions. It becomes a complicated business. So holding conversations which require eye contact, or admiring the view, while walking becomes extraordinarily stressful, as you are simply bending your mind to the task in hand: that is, not falling over. At times the logic of taking to a wheelchair seems overwhelming. Then, you enter another new world.

Chapter Ten

Italian Interlude

My first serious experience in a wheelchair was tempered by its context. We were having a short break in Florence with our friends Ruth and Anthony, in March 2004. Although Jane's great-great-grandmother had been an Italian lacemaker who, in Victorian times, had settled in London, Jane herself had never visited Italy, and my only encounter had been in my teens, travelling through from the old Yugoslavia across the north-east corner on the way to Switzerland and France. So this would be a first for both of us.

By now my mobility was evidently impaired. Access to aeroplanes and stairs would be difficult, as would walking long distances at normal speed. International air travel, however, turned out to be even more fun than normal. We were met at the terminal doors at Gatwick by an electric buggy, which whisked us and our baggage to the check-in, where I was transferred to a wheelchair, in which Anthony took me to the Club Class lounge for coffee until our flight was called. Then it was preferential treatment to the tarmac, up in the catering lift to the galley, and so to our seats. On touching down at Pisa the reverse process was carried out, Italian-style. I began to see a silver lining to my disability – not one which made it worth having, but something to be grateful for, nevertheless. In the enveloping darkness we drove through the Tuscan countryside and then down into the Arno valley, where the lights of Florence cast their glow into the night sky, and parked outside the Berchielli, our hotel overlooking the river. I went to sleep that night blissfully unconcerned about how I would get around to see the sights the next day. Fortunately, my companions were not so feckless and by breakfast had magicked an Italian wheelchair out of the management. There it was, silver and black, waiting for me in the hotel's marble-floored foyer. Pride reared its head. 'I don't want to be *pushed* round the streets of Florence. How undignified – among all this elegance!' But they were right. We would not get anywhere at my pace. And so my first experience of belly-level travel began, as we issued forth towards the Ponte Vecchio and the Uffizi.

In fact, if you could choose where to have your introduction to wheelchair life, I would recommend central Florence. It has a lot going for it. For one thing, it is on the level. For another, the surroundings are impressive. Almost every street is interesting, and every corner is exciting. The palazzo façades are tantalizingly beautiful; the piazzas are made for sitting in. If you can avoid the study-tour groups traipsing round the sites, the Florentines themselves have such élan and humanity. There is much to be said for sitting back and drinking it all in. What's more, they cater pretty well for the disabled, as we discovered when we reached the Uffizi, one of the world's great art galleries. We had heard that pre-booking was recommended, and we saw why. The queue, three deep, stretched back from the entrance a hundred metres. It would be a long wait.

But what was this? A ramp and a disabled entrance, with free priority access for the disabled and carer – and so we were in! (One had to learn to cope with the British guilt at jumping queues.) Although a wheelchair does not provide the ideal angle from which to view paintings, especially if you are short-sighted, it does at least prevent that tired-legged, totally understandable comment, 'How many *more* paintings have we got to look at?' which I heard from one member of a visiting school party.

One of my favourite sights in Florence was the side entrance to Santa Croce, the Franciscan church famous for its frescoes, including some by Giotto. The steps up to the front entrance make disabled access impossible, but there is a long ramp with a hairpin bend on the north side of the church, where there is a small door with a large notice above it: 'ingresso fedeli/believers entrance, ingresso disabili/disabled entrance'. If you want to pray in the side chapel, you can enter there without paying the tourist entrance charge; or if you are disabled they will allow you into the whole church. I enjoyed the juxtaposition – and the thought that this entrance was doubly intended for me.

Of course, there are places you cannot reach by wheelchair, such as the viewing gallery on the top of the Duomo, but there is so much else that this scarcely seems a hardship. The only drawback is the streets – not the traffic, as there is hardly any and what there is has no option but to give way to the overwhelming numbers of pedestrians – but many of them have small paving stones, or even cobbles, which provide a rough introduction to the joys of wheelchair travel. You bounce around, vainly gripping the armrests; your feet do a tarantella on the foot-plates and eventually fall off and stick out in front, waiting to be snapped off. You cannot protest; in fact, you can't talk at all, as your teeth are rattling. All you can do is surrender yourself to the experience and pray that your driver sees that approaching pothole in time.

The first lesson to be learned in a wheelchair is trusting the person behind it. You cannot tell how much they can see, especially at foot level, and you are all too conscious, in the crowded shopping streets of Florence, of the oblivious Achilles tendons in front of you, just waiting to be rammed by your metal footplates. You feel perilously close to them. You are on tenterhooks lest you fell a fashion model by her ankles, or run into an unamused mafioso. You desperately mouth 'Mi scusi,' being the only apology in Italian you know. Meanwhile, as your driver carries on animated conversation behind you, you wonder just how much they are concentrating on driving. The risk is compounded when your pusher is full of joie de vivre and kindly wants you to share it with him – as was the case with Anthony, who was sometimes like an inebriated gondolier on foot, indulging in episodes of 'Look, no hands!' down the steep streets of Siena. I found at such moments that laughing nervously, heavily disguised as nonchalance, and wildly waving my walking stick in the air helped to reassure the scattering Italians: 'Just some mad Inglese out for the day.'

The second discovery I made about being in a wheelchair in Italy was double-sided. On my side, I learned to accept help from strangers, and on their side, I found how consistently willing people were to offer help. My observation is that this was more so there than in England, and I suspect the reason has more to do with our culture of reserve than with national indifference. After we had visited Santa Croce together, Jane was pushing me back by the river and over the top of the double doors glimpsed one of those secluded courtyard gardens. From the wheelchair, the view was of blank rusting metal gate and stuccoed stone wall. It was early days in my wheelchair career, and so neither of us was very adept at extricating me. What's more, the brakes were not that efficient – in which case the wheelchair tends to shoot backwards as you try to stand up and you end up horizontal rather than vertical.

While we were struggling, a solitary passer-by noticed, crossed over from the far side of the road and helped me to my feet. I was rewarded by viewing an oasis of a city garden and by being reminded of the goodness hidden in human beings. He went on his way, and we did not see him again. I hope he had his reward too.

Then, sooner or later, you have to become accustomed to the well-known and annoying phenomenon, experienced by everyone with disabilities, often known as 'Does he take sugar?': the experience of suddenly becoming a non-person. You have not exactly become invisible, because you still feature in conversation, but you are more the object than the subject. That's when you really want to shout, 'Hello-o, I'm here, you know!' When a concerned-looking friend approaches and asks your carer, 'How's he getting on?' ... or a waiter asks your companion what you would like to eat ... or you are simply sitting there, at belly height, while a whole conversation (to which, what's more, you could – and would like to – contribute) carries on above your head... An extension of this is the law of diminished IQ. It is strange, but true, that there is a widespread belief that one's intelligence is located in one's legs. So the law of diminished IQ dictates that the more useless the legs, the less intelligent the person. Thus, if you have to talk to someone in a wheelchair, you must talk slowly and simply. It may help if you call them 'dear'. This law holds sway in many care homes up and down the country.

To be honest, I have not been that much troubled by the phenomenon, partly because of the increasing difficulty in my speech, which makes it understandable and helpful for those who know me well to interpret me, especially at parties, where there is so much background noise. However, there is one health worker whom I know and love who has never got the hang of it. To be fair, I am probably the first MND case she has dealt with, and I am sure motor neurone disease does not feature prominently on Dental Hygiene courses. But as I lie in that tilting chair from which there is no escape, I feel like a naughty boy being told off by his nanny once again. And when Jane arrives and I struggle to my feet, it seems as though the whole waiting room must hear the repeated injunctions. They are delivered slowly and clearly: 'I've told Mr Wenham he must brush right to the back on both sides. The gums are quite swollen. I've shown him this small brush, which will get right between the teeth. You can buy one from reception.' We mutter something about already having one, and I hobble round the corner on Jane's arm into the reception area. I feel curious pairs of eyes as I make my undignified entry: 'So that's him,' I feel them saying to themselves. 'I'd have thought he knew how to clean his teeth by now.' We confirm my next appointment and head for the door, as fast as I can. She is right, of course, and does an excellent job, so I'm grateful – through gritted but polished teeth. But I digress. Like me, she's from Tyneside, not Tuscany.

Back in Italy it was early days, and I cannot recall either invisibility or condescension there. Although it was mid-March, the sun came out on our last two days and the street cafés, where we sipped cups of dark glutinous chocolate, appeared with it. In the Piazza della Signoria we listened to a guitarist from Poland busking Bach and Rodrigo. In the evenings we dived into the bistros and wandered past the alluring shop windows back to the hotel. On Sunday morning at church, we found ourselves next to a woman who guided us through the service and translated the sermon. Her English was excellent; she ran a hostel for foreign (mostly American) students. Life was full and life was fun. After four days, we had one more sight to see before returning the hire car and checking in at Pisa airport for the flight to Gatwick. You would think, when you see pictures of the leaning tower, that it would be hard to miss; you imagine it dominating the city. The signs for the Torre Pendente looked promising. So we followed them and found ourselves in unremarkable suburbia: flats, garages, shops and traffic lights. It began to dawn on us that we had entered a concrete maze, from which, in the end, we were lucky to escape, making it to the airport via some back road with minutes to spare. I never did see the tower; not even from the window as the plane banked over Pisa. Our seats were on the wrong side. Oh well, 'Che sera, sera.'

Chapter Eleven

Emotional Incontinence

I am on my own. I am standing in the toilet next to my office, opposite the front door. Urine is running down my trouser leg and I cannot stop it. I feel so ashamed. I have been absorbed in work at home, answering letters, writing the monthly newsletter, or something. Time has slipped past. It is time for a pee. When I reach the loo, my bladder muscles suddenly spring to life. 'I'M NOT READY!' I silently shout to them, but they ignore me. I try not to panic, but I do panic. I struggle with the zip, all fingers and thumbs. Too late! The dark wet stain spreads down and reaches my toes. This time, as I am still able to, I remove trousers, pants, socks and shoes – when the flow has stopped – and sneak upstairs, hoping no one comes to the door just then. I clean up and dress, before Jane returns for lunch. I now understand why Dr Donaghy, on my last visit, asked whether I was having problems with incontinence. 'Oh, no!' I had blithely replied.

I had been more interested by my newly sensitized risible nerve. I had noticed a heightened tendency to find absurd things funny and to be unable to stop laughing. 'That,' he said, 'is a symptom of motor neurone disease. We describe it to our students as "emotional incontinence".' For me the term was immensely helpful, as it provided a handle for what could be both embarrassing and painful. I had never before experienced the acute side-splitting pain (which is just what I feel is happening) of uncontrollable laughter. It would erupt at predictable and unpredictable moments. Walking back from a Monday night committee meeting, a friend makes a witty comment and I am rolling in helpless mirth in the churchyard and up the path to our back door. Sitting at lunch, Charis, our two-year-old granddaughter, gives me one of the grins calculated to make me laugh, and my only remedy is to leave the room and take deep breaths. I have since learned that breath control is a vital tool in controlling this, and other kinds of incontinence; that, and avoiding situations of risk in the first place. Strategies such as not catching someone's eye, if you know they are high-risk. There are three hazardous individuals in our church, and I can't quite get over the old notion that hilarity and churches should not mix. Personally, I believe that churches should be places of unconfined joy; it is just that when people are queuing to receive the sacrament, fits of laughter are not helpful. (On the other hand, I have heard of a man performing cartwheels after receiving the bread and wine. Now *that* strikes me as appropriate.) So if I sense danger, regretfully, I avoid eye contact.

One of the major hazards is called Anne. She is one of the most life-affirming people I know. She has an infectious laugh and an infectious faith. I must not catch her eye if ever anything incongruous or amusing happens! Perhaps, therefore, it was no coincidence that, when I made my diagnosis public, she gave me the word 'Isaac'. She did not know that my mother's maiden name had been Isaac, but I doubt whether that was the point. Near the beginning of the Bible there is the story of Abraham and Sarah. They, we gather, are well advanced in years, way beyond retirement age, but have been promised a son. Not surprisingly, Sarah's reaction, much as she would have loved a child, is, 'You've got to be joking!' When, a few years later, the promised son is born – she must have been a tough old bird – they give him the name Isaac. Sarah comments, 'God has made laughter for me; everyone who hears will laugh over me.' The Hebrew word Isaac means 'he laughs'. Anne did not tell me all that, but as a sort of explanation added, 'The joy of the Lord will be your strength,' which is from a different story in the Bible. Joy? In the future, for me? Counter-intuitive and amazingly inappropriate in the circumstances, it might have seemed. Yet, for me, the reverse was true. Its effect was only positive, and it has proved true not only literally, but also in a profound and spiritual sense.

Not that it has been all laughs. Emotional incontinence cuts both ways, and I find myself vulnerable to romance, to grief and to deeply held convictions as well – all of which are liable to reduce me to tears. So romantic comedies are a dangerous cocktail. I have to hold my breath and close my eyes at crucial moments in Shakespeare to avert inordinate mirth or loud sobs, which might distract an entire theatre from what they have paid to see. Is it worth it, this living on a knifeedge? Why bother to expose myself to public embarrassment when we could as easily watch the plays on DVD at home? I blame the Royal Shakespeare Company, for putting on consistently brilliant – in our experience – productions and for being up with the Italians in catering for the disabled. Stratford is easily accessible for us, living in Oxfordshire, and once there we find they have reserved a parking space at no charge. Moreover, tickets for the disabled and their carers are *seriously* cheap. And anyway, to break out of the confines in which disease attempts to trap one is liberating for the spirit, even if physically taxing.

However, I suppose the effect of deeply held conviction is the least expected, but there it is: I am speaking about a great truth – for example, that love lies behind the universe, which I still believe – and emotion will spring like a lion and choke me. Or I am retelling Jesus' beautiful picture of the waiting father and the returning waster of a son, and there it is, surfacing again, that intolerable truth, 'God loves me' – and I cannot go on.

The fact is that much of life, as MND progresses, consists not of such highs (or lows, depending on your perspective), but of the mundane struggle to deal with the demands of survival. It is often said that this symptom of the disorder (lability) is inappropriate emotion. I tend to think of it more as unwrapped emotion. It is emotion uncontained. Out of the bottle. For someone as buttoned-up as I am, that's not entirely a bad thing, but I admit it does help if people know me! Those of us who have developed self-control to an unhealthy art form in the great English boarding-school tradition might benefit from a dose of lability, though I don't wish the disease on anyone.

By stealthy incremental steps, it has invaded all aspects of my existence. I have been fortunate in having one of the slower forms of the disease, as well as in having a highly competent full-time voluntary carer and excellent health professionals, from the beginning gently forewarning me what to expect.

My first speech therapist, Sue Bright, explained what was going on with my soft palate and my oesophagus, which would increasingly affect my speech and swallowing. She had me working on breathing from the diaphragm, and practising both that and the consonants which were presenting problems (such as a hard g), and gave me strategies for maintaining comprehensible speech, so that at the moment I am still able to take services and preach. According to those who know, MND does not affect the bladder and bowel muscles, and so I have no other excuse for advancing physical incontinence than the difficulty of getting to the toilet and then battling with buttons, zips and openings. But my experience is that I have lost some degree of control, a bit like Private Godfrey of *Dad's Army.* One day, I fear, it will not be so polite, and will confound my strategies to keep it contained, and I shall have to be catheterized, with a bag strapped to my calf. I guess that then I shall need that risible nerve. There's not much amusing about a catheter, or an incontinence pad.

Chapter Twelve

And So to Bed

One of the first gadgets that Lesley provided for me was the ambiguously named 'Bed Leaver'. I imagine some aspiring media studies graduate in product promotion being presented with this mysterious object and set the assignment to invent a name for it. What she would have seen is a plywood board some 20 centimetres wide and 50 long, with webbing straps metres long attached, and, at right angles, screwed in near one end, a metal hoop with a central pillar about 40 centimetres high. The best way I can describe it is: it's like a three-pronged fork – without the handle – stuck into this small plank of wood. She might well have been puzzled: 'How does it work? What's it for?' Its designer excitedly demonstrates. The board slips between the mattress and the bed frame. The straps fasten and tighten beneath the bed, leaving the hoop standing up next to the mattress, and there you have it: a ready-made handle which you can grab to turn over when lying down, or hold on to when sitting down, or lever yourself upright from prone, or push up on to stand up, from sitting on the edge, when you want to leave the bed. The graduate looks and listens. Then her eyes light up. 'Eureka! That's it! It has to be a "bed leaver"!' – nice pun.

When you become disabled, you enter a world of ingenious gadgets, some of which work better than others. This world can be accessed through the internet (search 'Disabled aids'), or catalogues sent by concerned friends, or of course those invaluable health professionals, such as physios and occupational therapists. One of my favourites is the long-handled toe and foot sponge: 'Ideal for cleaning the feet as well as between the toes without bending.' What you are not told is how you dry them afterwards. Then there is the long-handled sponge, exfoliating version, which 'has synthetic loofah on one side of the sponge head for added scrubbing action; also helps improve circulation' – and this is really nifty – 'The handle can be heated with a hair dryer and reshaped for those hard-to-reach areas.'

I once ordered from the internet what looked like being a neat device to attach to your trousers, so that when dropped they were not lost and out of reach for ever. When it arrived it turned out to be no more than two plastic bulldog clips attached to each other by string. The idea is, you attach one clip to your trousers and the other to your shirt *before* you let your trousers fall, and when you want to recover them, you just reel them in on the string. Simple, as long as securely attached, but worth £8? I'm not sure, but admittedly did find it useful with shorts in the hot July of 2006.

Lesley regularly checks up on what is becoming more difficult to manage. Sitting up in bed was one early casualty. I lost the necessary strength in stomach, leg and arm muscles and resorted to a laborious system of levering between bed-leaver and elbow; but it is fairly ineffectual, considering the effort. So she ordered a rope ladder for me, which I never really mastered. It is designed to help you sit up in bed. The ideal bed is one with a rail at the foot end; otherwise you have to make do with one of the legs. You tie one end of the ladder firmly to the foot of the bed and lay it on top of the duvet or blankets to within reach when you are lying down. When you need to sit up, you seize the ladder and, hand over hand, haul yourself upright. Hey presto, you're sitting up! That's the theory, I believe, but I did not take to it. Either I slid further down the bed as I pulled on it, or, when I let go, I soon fell backwards again. So I returned it.

That has been the fate of other devices, such as the bath board, to enable you to swing yourself safely into the bath, and the intriguing leg raiser. (Don't ask.) Talking of baths, they were one of the earlier casualties of the illness. One evening I found I couldn't get out. I couldn't draw my feet beneath me and the leg muscles were not strong enough to push up, so I just slipped to the tap end of the bath. From there I was rescued. My days of bathing were over. It would be showers from then on, with strategically positioned grab rails, to help in getting over the side of the bath and staying upright under the shower. Of course, the ultimate solution is a wet room with a roll-in shower, complete with seat. But that belongs to the era of stairlifts, or bedrooms on the ground floor, and I'm not quite there yet.

About a year into the illness, stairs were becoming more difficult. Lesley watched my progress up and down and foresaw the danger of my falling. So she prescribed a handrail to supplement the single banister. It might be aesthetically inelegant, but I did not fancy pitching head first down the stairs, even though, as Lesley reassuringly pointed out, it wouldn't be very far between landings. So she measured up and ordered metres of broom handle.

A few days later, the doorbell rang and I heard a familiar voice from the past. Brian Thomas is Welsh. He had been senior teacher and troubleshooter in Oxford, at my last school. You didn't mess with Mr Thomas. The last time we met had been more than twenty years ago. Now here he was, requisition order and toolkit in hand, on our doorstep. 'Well, I thought it must be you,' he said. He'd not changed much: same military moustache, a few more grey hairs, but considerably more relaxed. He had retired from teaching and taken on a management job with the firm which supplied and fitted medical and disability aids for our county. 'What's wrong with you, then?' He was never one to avoid the issue.

So I told him. He's the sort that is sympathetic without being sentimental. He went to the van to fetch the broom handles, which turned out to be poles about 5 centimetres in diameter. These stand away from the wall on metal brackets, meaning that you can grip right round them, giving you a firmer hold compared with the more elegant design which attaches directly to the wall. In fact, when I stained them to match the existing woodwork they didn't look at all bad. Before he went, Brian said, 'If you need anything else, just let me know.' And so it was I acquired my useful NHS walking stick, a week or two later, with the bonus of a renewal of an old acquaintance.

However, the bed leaver proved the surprising winner among useful devices. Without it, I flop on to the bed, heave my legs on board and lie on my back – and stay that way, like a stranded whale. I don't know what the subtle combination of muscle movements is that normally enables one to turn over without waking up, but I have clearly lost it. I clumsily thresh about with legs and arms and perhaps, if I'm lucky, manage to roll to my right, pushing Jane near the edge and of course waking her in the process. By then I am off my pillow and cricking my neck. Jane is wide awake. The only remedy is for her to push me back, at the risk of falling out of bed herself. But with the bed leaver I have much more leverage. I can manoeuvre myself from side to side, pull myself up and even roll over with more control. And it does live up to its name, in helping one get out of (and into) bed. As Lesley rightly points out, it is a matter of horses for courses. Aids work for some people and not for others.

Chapter Thirteen

To Sleep, to Dream...

Although the bed leaver works for me, it does not mitigate the problem of disturbed sleep. Whenever I need to shift position at night, I am woken up and have to work out what's required, whether it's an aching joint or a blocked-up nose, and how to achieve the desired relief, preferably with the minimum disturbance for Jane. I am fortunate in that I tend not to lie awake once I am comfortable (unlike Jane), but it has taken time to be reconciled to waking up six or more times a night, with accompanying dreams. It's a double bind. By the end of the day, you feel good for nothing except switching off and enjoying eight hours of oblivion. Your body says, 'Give us a break.' Yet instead of peace and sleep, you are wakened with regular irksome reminders of your condition. I realized of course that this was something I shared with millions of others, but it helped when I read Job, from thousands of years back, also complaining to God about this paradox:

> When I lie down I say, 'When shall I arise?'
> But the night is long,
> and I am full of tossing till the dawn...
> When I say, 'My bed will comfort me,
> my couch will ease my complaint,'

then you scare me with dreams
and terrify me with visions,
so that I would choose strangling
and death rather than my bones.
I loathe my life; I would not live for ever.

That is not poetic exaggeration. You are torn between welcoming and avoiding sleep.

When Hamlet said, 'To sleep, perchance to dream. Ay, there's the rub,' he was talking about dying and the possibility of a nightmarish afterlife in limbo or in hell. But I guess many MND sufferers would recognize the 'rub' of dreaming. I feel as though I have dreamed more in the past four or five years than in the whole of my life up till then. I realize that it is a factor of interrupted sleep, exposing the brain's subconscious activity, but it forms a vivid night-time life. Personally, I have had few nightmares on the terrifying scale in that time. However, I have frequently had the dreams in which I am fully fit again and enjoying hill walks and carefree days with my family. It's warm, and the sun is lighting up the fresh green of the water meadows. There's unseen standing water between the tussocks of grass and buttercups. The bedraggled dog bounces between the children, who are splashing ahead towards the gate leading up the hill and the bright beechwood which is our destination. Jane and I bring up the rear, massively content.

Or we are moving house. It's a new start. The house is in an Edwardian terrace, with steps up to the front door. We open it and begin an excited exploration. We show the children the rooms which will be theirs. They each have their own. We are in the long walled garden. On either side of the lawn there are established fruit trees. I can see our new neighbours peering at us from their back windows. Somehow, I can see into their gardens; they're neat and productive. At the bottom of ours is a vegetable plot, complete with compost heap and a door in the wall. It leads into a narrow road – or is it just an alleyway where discarded rubbish and shadows lurk?

The 'rub' with such dreams comes when I wake up, for one moment forgetting the disease or hoping that it has miraculously gone, until I try my heavy limbs and unresponsive muscles, and reality checks in. Nothing has changed. Another day of physical weariness and repeated frustrations has dawned. That night-time life was just a dream; *this* is the real world.

This is how Louise Halling, a woman aged twenty-eight who has muscular dystrophy, described it:

> I loved *Batman,* and I used to sit on my dad's knee and watch the show. The trouble was, I grew to develop a terrible fear of Catwoman, who I grew to believe lived under my bed, though why she should have chosen to live under *my* bed I didn't bother to question. I just knew she was there. So every night getting into bed became quite a challenge. I had to stand back about a metre from the bed and leap in under the covers in the hope that she wouldn't grab my ankle and

> pull me into her lair. Today sometimes I wonder when I wake up in the morning if I could just leap out of bed in a similar vein and somehow manage to jump past the lurking reality that is muscular dystrophy, then maybe I'd be safe, maybe I'd wake up and realize it was all pretend, it was just make believe, it was never there in the first place. But muscular dystrophy doesn't go away; it's an everyday disability; it's an everyday reality. Muscular dystrophy gets slowly worse over time.

Yes, the deterioration is relentlessly, mundanely, unglamorously real, stealing from you under cloak of darkness while tricking your mind with illusions. As time goes by, reality even invades those illusions, and in your dream world you are falling down hundreds of stone steps, or you find yourself being pushed in your wheelchair towards a cliff, and you can't utter a sound. Sooner or later, even in your sleep, you become aware that your body is failing.

Nothing is immune, not even sex. It does not take too much effort of the imagination to realize that the essential reciprocity of intercourse is undermined when one is reduced to wallowing like a beached whale. Not even a bed leaver can help then. How much longer will it be, I wonder, before I am unable to move my already clumsy hands and caress that beautiful skin with fingers already prone to cramp? In time will every means of telling Jane how desperately I love her be taken away? I know what the answer is. It doesn't help much to know it's the same for everyone. Why should it happen for Jane so soon? What consolation can I give her for all she gives me and does for me? And there's no denying I feel sorry for myself. For now, however, that does not mean an end to intimacy, nor indeed to shared joy together between the sheets. In fact such moments are more tender and more precious than ever. Jane makes me go as weak at the knees now as ever she did, and more so. The difference is, now it could have disastrous results if I were standing at the time. We might have to dial 999 to get me back on my feet.

The paramedics arrive. 'So, Mr Wenham, how did it happen?'

'Well, actually, she was just kissing me.'

Chapter Fourteen

The Slow Decline

Some gradients are imperceptible to the eye. You can detect them only when you are travelling on them, on a bicycle or, even better, in a wheelchair. The going is just that bit easier; it's not that you can freewheel, but you expend fractionally less effort, and little by little you lose height. You realize you are going downhill. With MND and similar diseases, the indicator is the reverse. Little by little, things become harder.

No one else notices. In fact, in their view it all looks plain sailing. 'I must say you look well,' they comment encouragingly when you return from holiday. No doubt it's true, and actually you do not feel inclined to moan, because you *have* had a great holiday and you *do* feel better for it. Yet at the same time you know that work is becoming fractionally harder; you can walk slightly less; eating takes a few seconds longer. When we were young it was a game to run up the down escalator and, as long as no killjoy adult turned us back, we could beat the countermotion. But now it is no game; it is all too real. And it is a constantly losing battle, for the force pushing you relentlessly down is within you, a fifth column betraying your efforts and undermining your strategies.

If you want to have some idea of what it feels like, Louise, with limb girdle muscular dystrophy, described the simple experience of walking better than anyone I know:

> I was diagnosed eight years ago, and since then it has got steadily worse. And although I look well – as everyone regularly tells me – I am an increasingly frequent wheelchair user, and I can't walk far without its aid, or the aid of crutches, provided that my hands are up to using them. I have muscles affected in my neck, shoulders, upper arms, wrists, hands, abdominals, hips, legs, ankles and, most embarrassingly, my buttocks, although the only benefit to that – as Mark [her husband] regularly tells me – is that I'm never likely to have to ask the question, 'Does my bum look big in this?'
>
> And I kind of struggle to explain actually what it's like to have weak and wasted muscles. But basically it's like this: most of the time I feel like I'm walking through sand, carrying a heavy back pack. With time the sand gets steadily thicker and the back pack gets heavier. I sometimes feel like I'm battling against a strong wind when I'm walking along the road, and I'm a little afraid of falling. I suppose I kind of feel that my life would be easier if there was someone there all the time physically holding me up, and I even fantasize about how much easier things would be if my whole body was wrapped in tubigrip. The fact that

I might look like an Egyptian mummy and sweat like a donkey stops me from actually trying it out.[1]

It's a matter of the thousand natural shocks that flesh is heir to, whittling away at one's system twenty-four hours a day, seven days a week. Five years ago I walked up Snowdon. Now, I need to pull on the handrails on both sides to drag my reluctant legs upstairs, and going down is a matter of minutes instead of seconds, as I cautiously balance each step of the way. It was balance that began to complicate dressing. At first it showed as a wobble when standing on one leg to pull on socks. So I would rest my back against a wardrobe. Then I had to sit down, and then physically place one leg on the other knee. Finally I could no longer reach my feet, to put on socks, or shoes, or trousers. For some time, by dint of fishing speculatively for a foot, I managed pants, but in the end even they defeated me, and now I have to rely on Jane in order to get dressed.

The most mundane things are in danger of becoming major and obsessive frustrations. The video and DVD players beneath the television gradually fell out of reach, so that I cannot change a film or a CD for myself. Anyway, removing one from the shelf or stack poses an increasing challenge, as they are inaccessible to my Rollator and without its support I would topple over, so moribund are my compensatory reflexes. Bottom shelves and bottom drawers are no-go areas, and the floor is a nightmare. Drop a paper or a remote control and it is gone for good until someone comes, and for the thousandth time I plaintively ask, 'Could you pick it up for me?' My perception is that those around me do not mind being asked, and neither do strangers, for the most part. My problem is my own pride. I do not like constantly to be making demands. No one likes a perpetual whinger. And surrendering my independence does not come easily; it makes me feel a failure. What good will I be soon? How much longer will I be earning my keep? Realistically, I am not economically viable now. The scrap-heap beckons.

Bitterness lurks. It's surprising how trivial are its triggers. A shoe is left in the way, a door is shut instead of open, the remote control is just out of reach, even the dog leaves her ball right where you'll step on it – and self-pity screams, 'Why don't they think?' To which reason replies, 'Do you really want them to live all their lives round your illness?' Of course I don't. As far as possible, I do not want to give the disease the satisfaction of interfering with my family's normality – including the dog's. So I try to put a mute in the mouth of self-pity, but I still occasionally catch it moaning: for instance, as it takes me so long to evacuate my bowels (or, more precisely, to get sorted afterwards), or as I find myself unable to reach a file I need to work on. There are hundreds of frustrations, and I know they will increase.

However, it is no good harbouring such negative thoughts. For one thing, such thinking is essentially self-indulgent and destructive; and, for another, it makes you a misery to be around. On 16 October 2006, BBC Radio Five Live's phone-in programme was on 'Who cares for the carers?'. Featured on it was a couple, Ned and Heather Cullen. Three years before, Ned had been flying Harriers in the Iraq war. Diagnosed with MND at the age of thirty-three, he now depended on Heather for everything: washing, showering, toileting, eating, moving, dressing. His form of the disease was much more rapid and was already more advanced than mine, so he had not had as much time as I have to adjust to its impact. Yet I was impressed, along with listeners and presenters, that neither he nor Heather was 'angry', which, as Ned commented in his extremely slow speaking voice, wouldn't do any good. It was more a matter of 'frustration'. 'We try to maintain a positive outlook on our life together.'

'Strangely,' commented Heather, 'it has brought us closer together, ultimately.' She was realistic, however, about the strains caused by the unpredictability of the progress of the disease and about the immense burden of emotional and physical tiredness. As the carer she had to be constantly aware of Ned's needs. Even at night in bed, she was conscious of the pattern of his breathing. I admired them immensely. They 'put life into perspective', said one listener later in the day, when interviewed again.

Keeping perspective as you descend further and further down the slope is no mean feat. It occupies more of your waking hours, because every task, from feeding to cleaning teeth, takes longer. At the moment I am fortunate in being able to eat more or less normally, but every mealtime is extended, as I have to be extra careful with each mouthful. My tongue is less adept at manoeuvring food around the mouth, my chewing action is slower, and my peristalsis, which I gather is the ripple effect of the muscles in the oesophagus moving the food down the gullet, has grown weaker. Choking while eating becomes a danger which strangers find quite alarming and to which family become accustomed. They are used to my spluttering and Jane's thumping me hard between the shoulder-blades (not officially recommended); but when we are out at a candlelit supper and I choke on a grain of rice, consternation runs round the table as I struggle for breath and try not to panic myself. Now, I know not to talk and eat at the same time. My parents would be proud of me: 'Don't talk with your mouth full.' (And I always thought it was because no one liked seeing a mouthful of half-chewed cabbage.) It's a matter of survival, but it takes time. So more of one's life is taken up with surviving and, almost inevitably, that dominates one's landscape. It's a long-drawn-out battle in which the forces against me gradually gain ground.

Note

[1] Louise Halling, talking at New Wine in July 2006, in the seminar *Growing with God through Hard Times.*

Chapter Fifteen

Thumbs Up

Quite often, people urge me not to give up. I don't intend to. I'm not inclined to surrender. As I have said, I know that I am comparatively well off in both the form and the stage of my illness. The symbol adopted by the Motor Neurone Disease Association is the thumbs-up sign, because it was the last communication David Niven gave before he died. It is well chosen, as my experience of patients has been of a similar spirit, like the Cullens'.

Without minimizing the struggle, it is not all frustration. Life is not an increasingly miserable decline. The landscape is not dominated by giants of anger and despair. They lurk nearby. Their shadows fall across your path from time to time, but you do not have to spend your time staring at them. You can enjoy other things on your journey.

For one thing, there's the fight itself. It is quite bracing. It is certainly purposeful. If you have taken the decision that you don't intend to cave in, then considerable energy and ingenuity go into surviving. Some things are ready made for you. Instead of trawling the internet for the latest armaments on the market to blow an enemy to smithereens, you look for the devices that will solve a problem or conserve your energy for a bit, and fortunately there are some well-informed salesmen and women (mostly the latter) to persuade you to try this latest gismo designed by a benign 'Q'. They will even, if you're lucky and it's not beyond budget, provide it for you. Actually, before rushing into internet shopping, you're well advised to talk to your health professionals (such as physios, occupational therapists and GP) and, if you have one, your local MND centre, who provide many aids without charge. Moreover, their advice is usually well-informed.

I took some time to latch on to the useful tips shared in the MNDA magazine and on their website. But you yourself also devise your own stratagems. Early on, when I began to need the banisters for stability, I simply carried books up and down the stairs in a carrier bag hooked over the wrist. I learned to avoid comfortable armchairs, as they seemed to become lower and lower and more and more difficult to get up from. Then I started to think ahead and plan the most energy-efficient way of doing things, from such trivia as not putting mugs away after washing up, as I would only have to get one out again next time I wanted a cup of coffee, to more major matters such as scheduling meetings at home. Some days I reach the end exhausted but satisfied; I may have been slow and clumsy, but I have achieved more than I expected. It's not been a bad day's work.

Moreover, you can learn to value slowness itself. It gives you time to appreciate life, frame by frame. Increasingly, contemporary life blurs by like a fast-forward effect on a film. We eat fast food and lose our sense of taste. We travel fast and lose our sense of perspective. We do not have time to listen to what someone else is saying. Our minds are in fast-forward. We hear what people say, but miss what they mean. Being slowed down and being capable of doing progressively less and less can be (and frequently is) frustrating. Yet it can have an astonishing effect.

As adults living in twenty-first-century Britain, we are invited to measure our value in economic terms. Success is rewarded and measured financially. Golden handshakes and productivity bonuses make some people very rich. But even away from the upper echelons of commerce, all of us get the message that we are valued for what we do, what we produce, what we 'contribute' to society. Unemployment is the ultimate negation of worth. In *The Full Monty,* the jobless miners make a great discovery: that they have a dignity, they're worth something, even when they are stripped bare.

Being inexorably rendered incapable is like undergoing an enforced, prolonged and embarrassing striptease. I can contribute less and less. I cannot even help to lay the table for a meal. The astonishing effect, however, I have found, is this: as I do less and 'just be' more, those nearest me, starting with my family, value me no less. Indeed, since my self-esteem used to depend in part on what I did, I feel that I am valued more. Their affection seems not to depend on my ability to meet their needs or to do anything.

First-century Christians had a word for this: *agapé.* It was the attribute of God, which is usually translated 'love' or, in the old version, 'charity'. Both English words have become debased through overuse. This is obviously an unusually gritty kind of love, as it does not hesitate to pick me up from the floor or to clear up my incontinence, and it strains and waits to understand my scarcely intelligible words. It clearly does not depend on my usefulness or attractiveness. The only explanation I can deduce is 'Because you're you.' I guess that is one of the most affirming conclusions someone can reach: 'I'm valued because I am me.' I admit I would rather discover the length and depth of such love by some other route, but I would be mad and infinitely sad not to appreciate it on the way. I have an inkling that it's more important than we dream.

It is paradoxical but true that slowing down gives more time. Instant communication has not brought the promised era of leisure, rather the opposite: a frenetic lifestyle, the modern dis-ease from which people dream of escaping 'to the country'. There the Super-Tramp, W.H. Davies, woos alluringly:

What is this life if, full of care,
We have no time to stand and stare?[1]

Well, to be brutal, MND is a sure-fire antidote to a life of frenzy, as doubtless are many other diseases. In a sense, it’s a case of one disease being a (drastic) remedy for another.

Note

[1] W.H. Davies, ‘Leisure’.

Chapter Sixteen

Cobwebs and Chickens

Enforced leisure has revealed things of surprising beauty for me. I never minded spiders, except the sort that jumped onto my bed at night in Kenya, and I can't quite understand why a friend should bring back a dead tarantula from Peru, but now I find them endlessly fascinating. I can sit and watch the epic explorations of a money spider for ages, as it lands on the breakfast table and sets off into uncharted lands between the cereal packets and the teapot, venturing over the edge of the world. 'What does it eat?' I muse. But it's the autumnal webs, glistening with dew and transforming the uniformity of the *leylandii* bushes with far more artistry than any Christmas tree ever carried, that really take my breath away.

When I was a child – typically, I imagine – I was fascinated by them: both by their delicacy and by their deadliness. It is a curious paradox, that combination of beautiful design and destructive intent, but, as some nature-programme presenters delight in graphically demonstrating, one that is replicated over and over again in the natural world. In our own part of that world, of course, we repeat the pattern, bending our best ingenuity and design skills to producing the means to destroy each other. Perhaps it was such thoughts that extinguished that childhood wonder; or perhaps simply the business of living. However, now I marvel as, propped between Jane and my walking stick, I pass the bushes with painful steps and slow in the early morning. It is not now the paradox that arrests my attention and entrances me; it is the infinite variety and sunlight-capturing beauty of these works of art hung with dew-drops, produced overnight not by designers trained at some art college, but by tiny instinctive creatures. And now I have the excuse – and the time – to stand and stare!

Behind the bushes where the spiders spin their webs lies another unexpected source of fascination: the chicken enclosure. Until the fox raided them there were six of them: six of the world's happiest hens. Not especially distinguished, they are Warrens, the common brown mongrels of the chicken world, or (to be more accurate) hybrids bred to be prolific egg-layers, but they have a good life – free to roam the small orchard behind our house in daylight hours, safely tucked up in their own ark at night. There were six, but not any longer. One decided to go AWOL, hopped over the wire fence surrounding the orchard and didn't return home to her sisters in the evening. We didn't find her; in fact, we didn't even know she was missing. But the fox, on his nightly patrol, sniffed her out, and in the early hours her desperate but short-lived squawking told us the whole story. There weren't even many feathers to show for it in the morning. Number two was our fault, as we forgot to pull up the ramp in the ark, which acts like a drawbridge. At midnight the fox called and unceremoniously seized the nearest leg on the perch. She obviously fought for her life, as the fox did not succeed in despatching her before my daughter, Rachel, and Jane arrived on the scene, scared off the fox and restored the hapless hen to her companions. However, there were many more feathers lying around that morning. And the post-traumatic stress permanently scarred her. Laying ceased. She would perk up for a time and then relapse into deep depression, having to be lifted down in the morning and spending days crouched motionless in the grass. She was not a happy fowl and in the end she had to go, despatched by our friendly gentle giant, Dave.

So now there are four. I could watch them for hours. Chickens are descended from guinea-fowl, I've been told, and their ancestors were forest birds. They certainly enjoy trees. They have their hiding places under the holly and hawthorn bushes by the garden wall, and outside our dining-room window, where I linger over lunch, stands their favourite apple tree. Their water container hangs from one low branch, and another is their chosen daytime perch. One, two or three of them will flap up onto it and preen themselves, or occasionally launch themselves, as a lumbering and easily dodged missile, at a sparrow pecking in the dust below them. Once or twice all four have managed to squeeze onto it in peaceful coexistence, but not for long. Usually the others make life on the branch subtly uncomfortable for the fourth, and down she flutters in indignity. I imagine, but don't know, that it is always the same bird that falls, and presumably she is also number four in the famous 'pecking order'. There is no sentimentality among our hens; number three is quite gratuitous in her pursuit of four. (Our first six hens each had names, from Tonight to Bob the Pigeon, for reasons too convoluted to explain, but their successors can count themselves lucky with numbers.) When they gather round the cylindrical food hopper, there is plenty of space for all four, and they move together in a clockwise direction as they feed; but Three goes out of her way to take vicious pot-shots at her sister Four's head. The latter seems to take it in good part and merely slots in on the other side between her two other sisters, who do not seem to mind. Presumably they are less insecure than Three. Four was the only one to undergo the indignity of an autumn moult, looking as though she'd had a narrow escape from a plucking machine – a tousled, tatty bundle of brown and white and the butt of ridicule from her sisters. But now, she has a sweet revenge. Her comb is bright red and her coat a stunning, sleek gingery number reminiscent of fox fur. She is simply the belle of the roost.

Apart from these occasional spats, however, it is a harmonious little community out there. I watch them when they sense danger and all four, like avian meerkats, wherever they are, stand motionless and point in the same direction – until they relax and return to grubbing around in the grass. But very little threatens their safety, aside from the fox's night-time visits. United they stand, and if a cat should wander into their enclosure they will face it off. In the summer I watch them basking in the dips they have created, which are so deep that it has become impossible to mow the tussocks that are left. When it is *really* hot, they do the chicken equivalent of panting, while holding the wings partially open to let the fresh air get to their 'armpits'.

I watch them preening each other and themselves with their amazing, rubbery ET necks, which let their beaks reach parts of the body that are beyond the conception of someone who has trouble turning his neck even as far as 90 degrees. They are constantly on the move: scratching in the earth, chasing daddy-longlegs and rushing from all corners, in a headlong mixture of flying and running, to the window whenever it's opened, in the hope of some scraps coming their way. They have such an incredible, comic design. I dare say it has been caricatured in the process of crossbreeding, but that ungainly fat ball of feathers on spindly horny sticks of legs has no business to be flying, or running for that matter. Yet they defy augury and succeed in both. I envy their effortless balance when they stand on their branch on one leg while scratching their necks with the other – without even a wobble! They are endlessly watchable, strangely beautiful and even endearing. And, of course, they produce real free-range eggs, particularly

Four, who produces bigger, browner eggs than her tired sisters. As I linger after a meal, I sit and stare – and reflect that I'm lucky to be able to do so.

Chapter Seventeen

French Interlude

Cobwebs; chickens; and then there was the evening of the crickets (or were they cicadas?). Not in England, of course, but in the Charente region of France, near the medieval village of Aubeterre, beloved by modern tourists – nearest airports Bergerac and Bourdeaux, to give some sort of geographical fix on it. It is the late summer of 2006, unseasonably cool for the month of August, and we are on holiday with an extended family group in a large converted barn, where we have all met up for a week. In fact Jane and I have not flown, as I now have too much equipment to lump around with us – wheelchair, Rollator, shower seat and toilet seat, in addition to normal luggage. It would simply be a nightmare for Jane. So we have taken the fast ferry and driven via disabled-friendly bed-and-breakfasts down the west side of France. We have enjoyed the adventure, which to my relief has been incident- and accident-free.

I'm relieved because we were unable to obtain insurance cover for me. There *are* firms who will provide reasonable cover for MND sufferers (about whom the MND Association provides details – along with the stricture that it is essential to have insurance when abroad). As part of the application process one is referred to a medical screening company who, either on line or by telephone, ask you about your condition. I was doing fine until asked about any other chronic conditions. When I mentioned epilepsy (albeit inactive for more than six years), I was declared uninsurable. The other big mistake, I gather, is to describe one's condition as terminal. Thus we were presented with a dilemma. Should we ignore the experts' advice and travel nevertheless, relying on the partially useful European Health Insurance Card; or should we cancel and let down everyone else? Sometimes we experience amazing kindness, and when we were debating this was one such occasion.

I mentioned in a church home group that we were concerned about this, as one does among friends who pray. Some days later, one of our church members stayed at the end of a service and said, 'We [she and her husband] would like to be your insurance cover for your holiday.' I was aware that the implications of the offer were immense, and I knew that they were also aware. They would stay contactable by phone the whole time we were in France; they would be prepared to come out and bring us back to the UK if we were stranded; and, most open-ended of all, if I ended up in hospital and with escalating medical costs, they were prepared to bail us out. This couple are by no means millionaires, but are among the richest in spirit that I know. I have often preached about God's grace and the fact that his greatest desire is that we simply accept it. Now, faced with human grace, I had an inner struggle, but really knew that I had no option but to say, 'Thank you.' So, armed with our EHICs, insurance for Jane and cover from our friends, we had set out.

Now, after nights in Normandy and the Loire and days of leisurely travelling, we are ensconced in our isolated holiday let. It has been one of the few warm days. The grandchildren are in bed. We have enjoyed – yes, enjoyed – one of those hackneyed 'the English in France' meals on the vine-surrounded terrace, lingering over our wine and coffee, with drifting conversation. We look out over a meadow running down to a stream and a wood stretching left and right as far as the eye can see, from which occasionally deer may emerge and then merge back into the shadows. We gather from Frank and Chris, our hosts, that *sangliers,* wild boar, also inhabit the surrounding woods; in fact, one was killed in their field by the local hunt not long ago. The *chasseurs* are so trigger-happy that if you go walking at the weekend you are wise to wear a luminous hat, to avoid becoming a trophy on someone's wall. But this evening all is peaceful. The sun is gradually sinking towards the hills on the other side of the valley, and as its rays cease to reach us, we notice the chill of the breeze. However, we are reluctant to take refuge indoors. Though we don't know it, the show is just beginning.

Above the hills the clouds, which hitherto seem to have had a running battle with the sun to intercept its warming rays, have now become the principal subject of the ever-changing canvas which it is painting in front of our eyes. We sit in companionable silence, admiring something so much more subtle and beautiful than any kaleidoscope, imperceptibly shifting hues of rose, and orange, and purple, and blue – though no words, nor paints either, can do justice to the unfolding variety before us. And meanwhile, near to us, the grass and the trees are darkling, as they fall deeper and deeper into shadow. Then, from below, somewhere in the wood, a cricket starts up his stridulation, that repetitive yet never tedious song amazingly produced by the rubbing together of wings. It's not long before he is joined by another, and then another, and soon all along the woods below and in the trees behind us there are crickets chirruping, each with his own call, none identical, stretching away into the perspective of distance. This is not a Grand Canyon or Victoria Falls spectacular, but it is nevertheless spectacular: a moment of beauty which does not last for long, but which reaches deep. It is worth lingering over. Together we savour the symphony of sight, sound and affection, until in the cool night air my muscles begin to seize up. But the memory and the mystery remain.

Such moments, whether dew-spangled spiders' webs or cricket-loud sunsets, are, I think, an intimation of immortality. We can analyse the mechanisms and processes of what we experience, but the wonder with which we are filled is nothing if not worship, either for the thing itself or for its source. Or we may settle for a baser admiration of our own cleverness in understanding, explaining or putting it on show for others, as in the extra bits in wildlife films showing how it was all shot. The privilege I now enjoy is time to enjoy the beauty all around me, to which occupation made me blind, and for that I thank ... Whom? Or what? A young friend of mine once memorably described the beauty of the natural world as the 'hem of the Creator's garment'. I like that. It implies that we see only the fringe of the beauty inherent in its source; that the lesser comes from the greater. There is an even greater beauty waiting to be found. It also implies a potential for healing. The phrase originates in the story of the diseased woman in the Gospels who says, 'If I may only touch the hem of his [Jesus'] garment, I shall be healed,' which indeed she is. In harmonious encounter with the natural world's beauty we experience something akin to the restorative potential of music; something that settles our spirits and hints at an ultimate Beauty.

To put it more mundanely, in the sentimental film *Fifty First Dates,* after a motor accident the main character suffers long-term memory loss. In fact she can remember only the events of the current day. Every morning she wakes up with her memory wiped clean. This presents a problem for the man she falls in love with. She doesn't ever recall meeting him before, presenting him with the conundrum of how to progress the relationship. So they keep having 'first dates'. The line from the film which struck me recently when I first saw it on television was, 'There's something special about one's first kiss.' When living in the shadow of death, every day is a new day of life: a day to experience the kiss of the sun, the caress of affection and the beauty of your whole world again, yet with a first-time ingenuousness. There's something special about the first day of the rest of your life.

Chapter Eighteen

Travelling Companions

The company on the journey is special, too. I love it. Maybe my growing social ineptitude makes me more tolerant or appreciative of others. Maybe this is also a factor of time. Not being able to rush about means having more time to take notice of people. Maybe it comes from being toppled from my professional pedestal as a 'people person' to being just another person. In the media, clergy are often portrayed with derision – witness Rowan Atkinson in *Four Weddings and a Funeral* – but that may reflect the residual superstitious respect with which we are still commonly regarded. I remember one redoubtable Stockport widow's Thatcheresque reaction to being told that the new curate was shy: 'Well, he has no business to be.' No, the myth is that clergy are a race apart: socially adaptable, morally irreproachable and, above all, 'religious'. And although the enlightened chattering classes know it to be a myth, yet they still feel a compulsion to create ridiculous caricatures and to revel sanctimoniously in a priest's 'fall from grace'.

However, it's different when God apparently knocks one off his perch. I'm no longer articulate; it takes me a long time to form my sentences, and I need to choose words that are easy to say. I feel frustrated at my inability to nuance my ideas. I am in danger of losing abstract expression and talking only of the day-to-day. I'm no longer mobile. I cannot get out and about on my own; I can't go visiting. I can't participate in meetings. I'm a dead loss socializing. It is not a matter of being shy. It is more a matter of being useless. Which, for some people, is reassuring, as here at least is one man of the cloth who poses no threat. For others, it is rather puzzling. Why, for one thing, does God have such pathetic representatives? More down to earth, how does the Church justify employing me? I must admit, it puzzles me. As long as four years ago, I was in tears. I wrote:

> Every day my flesh says, 'Give up. Buy a bungalow and retire.' The simplest things are an effort. The most mundane take an age – walking to church needs ten minutes. Were it not for Jane, I'd go barefoot, unfed and be housebound – and be no use to the parish. I'm told I'm needed...

Later that week, my friend Gareth called round. He is from Yorkshire and is a vet; his wife is a consultant paediatrician and is from Lancashire. Between them, there's not much they miss about one's physical state. Gareth and I had regular duels on the squash court, where my speed was matched by the weight of his punch. I suspect that he and Barbara were the first in our church to recognize my early symptoms and what they indicated. I remember during the time of my hospital tests, when we were driving to the leisure centre for a game, Gareth asked me what was going on and I told him about the tests and the possibilities. His reply was the epitome of sympathy and Yorkshire bluntness: 'Oh, bugger.' There was not much more to say, and I dare say we worked out what was unsaid on that uncomplaining squidgy black rubber ball. With my advancing MND our squash fell into decline and ceased, but I asked him and Barbara to be among the handful of people who knew me well enough to say, 'We think you should stop working now.'

Gareth himself was increasingly plagued by a bad back, which made large animal work, his speciality, unsuitable for him. So now, with a school-age family, he was considering difficult decisions about his future. Although we talked about that, his main message was, 'We think it's time for you to call it a day.' I logged the verdict, both in my mind and on paper. A day later there came a unique (to me) delivery to our door. It was from the Channel Islands: a bouquet of flowers with a rainbow variety of colours and a message, from a student who had visited us a year before, that we were being remembered.

I did not then call it a day. I decided to keep going. However, Gareth's breath and honesty were not wasted. There's a proverb, 'Faithful are the wounds of a friend.' In one way, it hurt to hear a clinical judgement that I was no longer competent to carry on. I knew it was neither lightly arrived at nor given as criticism. It came from friends whose primary concern was our quality of life. But in another way it came as a relief and a release. I had permission to stop struggling. It would be no disgrace or defeat if I were to resign. Ironically, as a result, lightness has entered my working life, as I no longer stay in post out of duty but out of choice.

Friendship comes from unexpected directions. I never found out how our postman came to know about my illness. Presumably it was talked about in the village post office; most of what happens around the area is discussed there. But there was no necessity for Paul to knock and to bring the post to where I sat at my desk. No one told him how hard it was becoming for me to pick the letters up from the hall floor. We didn't waste much time, but it was a gesture of kindness and a contact in my solitary mornings when Jane was out, both of which I found significant. Thus I was not a little put out when Royal Mail's powers that be chose to reorganize our local rounds and Paul was sent elsewhere. He had been more than a deliverer of the post. I must say, from where I sit, that sort of service is worth a great deal of 'efficiency' and 'cost-effectiveness', even though Royal Mail's management has a different perspective, I gather.

However, it did not turn out as I feared. After a period of discontinuity, when we never knew who would deliver the mail from day to day, nor when the letters would land with a dull thud on the mat, we eventually settled to two main posties. Sue, our regular, and Simon, her husband, who share our round, have proved equally friendly and helpful. When I am on my own, again unasked, they have taken to bringing the post right in to me. It is obviously more than they are required to do. There is simply a degree of care there, which makes life better.

I am of course not the first to have noticed the way in which others' misfortunes release compassion in people. The utopian conundrum is this: if we were to be able to eliminate all suffering from the brave new world, would human compassion wither and disappear? And would such a compassionless world be better than our present mess? I am not arguing against the relief of suffering, or medical research, or the relentless pursuit of peace. Of course not. At the best, they are motivated by defiant compassion. However, I do wonder whether we fairly weigh the cost of the current consensus that disease, pain and death are unmitigated – even absolute – evils.

Paul Brand, the great leprosy surgeon, first alerted me to the beneficial side of pain. He pointed out the simple fact that the disfigurement and disability of leprosy sufferers were caused not directly by their disease, but by the deadening of sensation in their limbs. The result was that they were unaware of, for example, the heat of fire, and so easily got burned. Without the defence mechanism of pain, we are vulnerable to the physical forces of the universe. In that sense, pain is good. Naturally, such a brave new world is an unattainable dream. So maybe the conundrum needs no answer. And a further question I find myself asking can certainly not be answered here: 'Is there compassion in heaven?' Or, to be more precise:

'If there'll be no suffering in heaven, will there be any compassion?' Perhaps it needs to be the subject of its own book. (I hope that I'm not evading the issue. For me – and, I have found, for many facing their own or another's death – it is an important question and a real one. Yet for many others, I know, it's a non-question, and I don't want to lose half my readers now!)

I have never met some of my fellow-travellers, but I recognize them when I hear them. Louise Halling is one of them. Angela Beise is another. She is a mother, living in Paris, whose son Michael has multiple handicaps resulting from a rare genetic syndrome, 18Q-minus. Recently I read her account[1] concerning their search for a specialist school for him. Because waiting lists were so long, it was suggested they try a school for Down's syndrome children, even though Michael does not have Down's. Down's schools, she was told, were taking children with other syndromes, because testing in early pregnancy meant that fewer parents were choosing to complete the pregnancy. So fewer Down's children are being born. Reflecting on her reaction of shock to this statement, she writes:

> Michael has benefited greatly from the incredible advances in medical technology. He was born with a cleft lip and palate, and feet that required extensive surgery. I am grateful for the amazing doctors, and technology, that have so beautifully met his needs. But today I wondered whether

> technology was robbing us of an important element of society.
>
> In the days that followed I tried to imagine a society void of disabled people. What if this technology reaches a stage at which any or all babies with special needs can be eliminated? What would society look like if everyone were 'normal', if we never had to make provision for people who are slow, or deaf, or blind, or lame, or crippled? What if we could eliminate the 'weak' altogether? The question that haunted me was this: Do disabled, imperfect people contribute anything to society? Do we need them to be balanced, healthy and whole?

Her answer begins with her own family:

> My children are among the most selfless, giving people I have ever known. I am in awe of them. They have made sacrifices, too numerous and too big to calculate, for their handicapped sibling. One might think that this would make them bitter and discontented with life. In fact it has done exactly the opposite. They are thankful and giving, and tolerant of difficult and unlovely people. Could it be that these 'imperfect' people somehow balance society as a whole?

Note

[1] In Anita Cleverly, *Destiny's Children* (Kingsway, Eastbourne, 2005), pp.190ff (reproduced with permission).

Chapter Nineteen

The Fellowship of the Road

One way or another, there are a lot of us on this road, involuntarily. What makes it more tolerable are those who *choose* to walk it with us, not because they have to but because they want to; not because they can take the road away, but because they want to be there with us. This fellowship of the road has extraordinary power. There is a mystery about it which beggars analysis. I do not know why friendship assumes such significance in pain, of whatever kind, but it does. The film *Cold Mountain* is full of friendships forged in the face of horrific suffering during the American Civil War, and for me the triumph in the story lies in the quality of those diverse relationships. Ruby walks into the life of Ada, the dead preacher's daughter, at her lowest point, trying and failing to survive on her own. 'I know your plight,' Ruby says. She does not want to be paid; just to share her life. 'I expect to board and eat, at the same table. I ain't a servant, if you get my meaning.' And so the practical, earthy labourer's daughter comes alongside the airy, book-loving Ada, and a bond of friendship grows up, which transforms them both and carries them through a purgatory of pain and fear to a springtime of content.

So who has chosen to travel with me? Who are my Rubys? Choosing comes either in opting in or in not opting out. Some have made the deliberate decision to join me and others have equally deliberately decided to stick with me, even though both come with a cost. Foremost among the latter are my family, as well as a surprising number of friends. Among the former are two couples, Anthony and Ruth, who have already played a part in this story, and Charles and Mandy, who moved nearby in 2001.

We walked into Anthony's and Ruth's lives when Paul, our eldest son, proposed to their elder daughter, Penny. Unpredictably, the new in-laws hit it off well together. As far as busy lives and homes more than a hundred miles apart allow, we would count each other as friends. However, within a year of the wedding my MND was looming on the horizon, and soon after its diagnosis Ruth and Anthony came to stay with us. During the visit they made a commitment: 'We will stand with you through this whole thing.' And so they have. They are our most regular visitors and holiday companions. We laugh together – often. We also feel safe enough to weep with them – and we do. We have shared all of our lives, from family to food. Most of all, a deep friendship has taken root, which we know will last, even outliving death.

Charles and Mandy walked into our lives by a different route. They make an unusual couple. Mandy is an artist who paints visionary pictures. She is readily recognizable by the pink streaks in her hair, which in some way reflects her personality. Charles, by contrast, appears more conventional. Always smartly dressed, with a well-trimmed beard, he has an almost military bearing. From an uppercrust family, public-school educated, he went from a career in the City of London into ministry in the Church of England, until taking early retirement and buying a former flour mill. He and Mandy had a vision for transforming it from its half-converted state into a beautiful home, where you can see the mill-race flowing underneath, with the outbuildings and surrounding land creating a peaceful haven hidden unpromisingly behind a service station. The peace is occasionally disturbed when a rainstorm swells the brook and brings with it a succession of natural and man-made detritus which threatens to clog up the mill stream. Then Charles dons a pair of waders, stands in the racing water and extracts anything from trees to traffic lights. If he is not there, then Mandy takes the plunge. They were defenceless, however, against the summer floods of 2007, which swirled through and around the buildings and devastated the ground floor. And so, taking a deep breath, they set about restoring and improving their original design.

They were completing the work for the first time when Charles went to see the bishop about permission to take services in the area (a 'licence to officiate', in Anglican-speak). The bishop suggested that he might have a ministry supporting me. Our first meeting –

in fact, we had lunch together – happened two days after we had heard my diagnosis. Immediately we knew that this was meant to be. There was instant rapport, and we had so much in common.

These were people with whom we could be real. They knew how to help those in trouble. They had faced their own most terrible tragedy, when their infant son died in a house-fire. Theirs is no cheap sympathy; it is above all full of faith and hope. That lunch set a monthly pattern which continues as a vital feature of our calendar. With them, as well, we are able to be honest; in fact, it is quite hard not to be, as Mandy has the knack of asking the intuitive probing question. When one afternoon she asked me, 'So would part of you like to be released?' it was as if she had unblocked a pent-up stream of frustration and hurt, and suddenly a placid stream became a swirling torrent, for a time – which was of course ultimately healing.

Travelling with me comes at a cost: a cost which I am scared to ask anyone to pay. Angela Beise says this about bringing up a disabled child:

> To parent a disabled child will require many ambitions to be laid aside... The child will become the focus of most of your time and energy and will determine what you can and cannot do in many situations. He can bring limitations to the dreams you can pursue. He can bring more sleepless nights than most parents will ever have to endure. Parenting seasons will be unusually

> long, and grief will last the lifetime of such a child. Parents not only grieve the child they 'lost' at his birth but grieve as they watch him struggle with tasks that normally come easily to a child of his age. They grieve when he realizes he is not like other children, and when they see him in physical or emotional pain...

However, after all that, she concludes:

> I am one parent of a child with special needs who is better because this child came into my life. Would I have chosen this road? Never in a million years. Am I grateful for the changed person I am today? You bet. Would I trade one sleepless night, hour in a hospital, penny spent on medical bills, or minute in a therapist's office? No chance. All heartache considered, I'll take the imperfect society.

In my case, the cost for those who care for and about me is the certainty of watching the grim deterioration of someone whom they are not keeping at arm's length, let alone out of sight and out of mind, and of impending devastation in loss. I cannot tell whether they will be able to echo gratitude for the road they have walked with me. I have no doubt that never in a million years would they have chosen it. I can speak of the journey only from my side. Well, to be honest, I can't, because it goes beyond words. The deep-down tenderness and matter-of-factness of my family amaze me. I have a wife, four adult children and a daughter-in-law. In the autumn of 2005 they were all home for a family celebration. A few days afterwards I wrote:

> Celebrated Jane's birthday a week late, with all the family here. I get such deep joy from seeing them all and their being good friends. And from their faith and gentleness. I suppose the one thing I have to fight against is the feeling of guilt which I can sense in me, for landing them with a dad and a husband who is a cause of pain to them. I know they hate seeing me deteriorate, and pray for my healing...

Most of the time the grief is hidden, but sometimes it surfaces, momentarily, which is fine. Yet we have never had a good family bawl. Perhaps it would help, but our consensus is that it would not. Where there is sufficient empathy, the merest signal speaks volumes. The nearest we came to a shared blow-out was Christmas Day 2003, when I felt the need to talk about the future, which seemed to me imminently precarious. I did not succeed in speaking coherently, but quite effectively spoiled what we look forward to as a highlight of our family year. Was it a foolish thing to do, at an emotionally charged season of the year? I thought so at the time, and yet a family needs to face pain together and to communicate it. And feelings run deeper than polite rational discourse can always express. It was certainly foolish in this sense, as I have discovered and should have known, the future is neither certain nor in our hands.

More often we enjoy the normality of life. Laughter is common currency when we are together – not the hollow laughter of the jester defying the darkness, but the warm laughter of companionship on a shared journey. There is no denying it's a puzzling journey for us all. It's an enigma how we come to be travelling it. There is no history of MND in the family to suggest it might be genetic. There is no other identifiable 'cause'. It is a mystery when or where it will end. It just happened one evening, in 2002, I told my family that I had tickets for them to come with me on this grim mystery trip – and none of them then or since has said, 'Actually, Dad, I don't much like this journey, and I'm going to get off. Hope you understand.' Nor has Jane hinted, 'This is so much worse than we bargained for. I'm out of it.'

I remember the founding of Helen House, the children's hospice in Oxford and the first of its kind in the country. At the time I was teaching just round the corner in Cricket Road, at the former Cowley St John Upper School. It was acknowledged to be a tough school with a complete mix of students, but they all liked and had respect for Sister Frances Dominica, the slight, gentle figure in blue and white who came to talk about her vision for terminally ill children. She smiled a lot; she spoke quietly – and they listened. With the passing of many years, she, if anyone, should understand the situation of both the children and their parents. The bewilderment and the agony defy imagination. She still visits schools to talk about the work she began. I guess her message is still the same.

> We can't change the world, but actually, in very small ways, we can change the world, because we can make a difference in our lives, maybe to one person, but a profound difference; just by coming alongside, by walking a bit of their journey with them, not having the answers, but having the courage to stay in the unknowing with them. That's what friendship is, I think.[1]

You'd better believe it. That has been my experience.

Usually I enjoy navigating as well as driving. From my point of view, I like to know the route plan and to be master of my own destiny. Now that neither is true, what makes the land of unknowing bearable for me is my final travelling companion, the ultimate in friendship. (I hesitated to write that, for fear of it seeming too trite or too flippant, but can't find truer words to describe the heart of the matter. It's more personal than an ideology, and yet beyond a person.) I believe that God has not given up on me, and *de facto* knows both the destination and the route. I can't prove it, but for me the evidence is there. Therein lies my ultimate security. In mountaineering terms, He's both guide and anchor man.

Much as I enjoyed hill walking, I have never done serious mountain climbing. The idea of going the hard way up a peak never appealed to me. If there were a choice of railway, path or climb, I'd choose walking the path over the railway. But the idea of clinging to some sheer cliff face, dangling on a rope held by someone perched scarcely less precariously above me, seems foolish. My grandfather was a considerable Alpine climber, and I suppose I had heard from him of the White Spider on the north face of the Eiger. When I saw it for myself as a teenager, I could grasp why it was such a legend, that permanent pattern of ice on the sunless, seemingly vertical mountain face. Neither love nor money would have tempted me near it. Now, on a mountain of a different sort and not of my choosing, curiously, I have no fear of falling or dropping into a bottomless crevasse. There is a rope which will hold me, even if I lose my grip. That's enough knowing for me. When the rope goes taut and I reach the end of it, I don't think I'll be disappointed.

Note

[1] *The Children of Helen House,* BBC2, 9 January 2007.

Chapter Twenty

Briers and Roses

The week my MND was finally diagnosed, before anyone outside the family knew, someone from the village called round. 'I felt God telling me to give this to you,' she said. I knew her quite well, but this was a unique but characteristic occurrence. She had come across a book on a second-hand bookstall, of which she already had a copy. I looked at its title. It was *Rose from Brier.* It seemed uncannily apt. It was written in 1950 by a well-known Christian missionary in South India named Amy Carmichael, whose writings verged on the mystical. I thanked Jules, but did not tell her why it might have been timely. It might well have stayed on my desk, gathering dust, had it not been for the following Sunday.

That was the day when I had emotionally broken my news to the church in the morning service. In the afternoon my brother from Oxford drove over to see us. He had brought me a plant, a unique gesture but not uncharacteristic – well, you do, don't you, when people are ill? It was a miniature rose, in bud and in flower. Some would call it mere coincidence; some would call it providence. For me it was a promise that pain and sweetness could grow together. And it suggested that I was not alone, adrift on a malign and meaningless sea. There were some stars showing through the clouds. Later we planted the rose in the garden, where it still flowers each year.

It is such small incidents that begin to form what I previously described as the 'evidence' that God is on the case. I keep what's known in the trade as a spiritual journal, though rather an erratic one. It is a cross between a diary, a commonplace book (with resonating quotations) and my own reflections. I began it when radically impacted by an experience of the Spirit, which I did not want to forget. From October 2002 it becomes a rollercoaster, recording swoops down into grim introspection and unforeseen switchbacks into joy. Much of the evidence is recorded there.

> Hi ... I felt I had to email but it's quite difficult. I don't want you to feel intruded upon. My Mum and I were praying for you and your family this morning and Mum got a picture of Jesus looking in complete compassion, with arms outstretched, over you and your family and the words 'My children suffer not in vain'. She gets these things quite a lot, and hopes it can be an encouragement for all of you.

This came in an email to my son, Stephen, in April 2003, from a friend who had been at university with him but never met me. She sent him another at the beginning of January 2004, a few days before I crawled off the pavement up the pub drainpipe and was paralysed by the fear of falling in the churchyard. 'Mum's had another picture while praying... She had a picture of Jesus standing in the centre of your parents holding their hands. Then this morning she also had the words "In me abide. Be at peace." She hopes this is timely and helpful.' Uncannily timely!

In November 2004, I wrote:

> it had been a couple of bad days with my being gloomy about whether I'd really be any use staying on here. Tuesday morning for some reason had the idea of taking coffee up to the Ridgeway, where Jane walked and I wrote letters... It proved a day of recreation. That afternoon Karen rang from her home in West Palm Beach in Florida. She had woken at 4 am (9 our time) with the urge to pray for us.

Karen is an international intercessor (someone who prays for situations round the world). She had once stayed with us to pray for our area, but we don't have contact except for the occasional email. One might make no connection between the coincidence of a change of mood in me and a prayer in America followed by a telephone call, but the conclusion I reached then was, 'God does know and care.'

In my journal there are recurring moments of doubt, usually about whether I should still be in the job. It is an unusual job, since I am in one of the anomalous (for these days) posts which has 'freehold'. That's basically security of tenure until retirement age, barring some gross misdemeanour. In principle, I could be an utter liability and still retain my job. Some people probably think it's already the case!

Fortunately we also have a regular review process, which involves being assessed by church members, professional colleagues, an independent assessor and the boss, who in my case is the bishop. It is, in theory, meant to affirm and help your professional development, but of course it feels as though you are being scrutinized and held to account. It can be crushing. However, it does provide a reality check for overweening arrogance, as well as for cripplingly lost confidence. My review came late in 2005. The conclusion was that I should be continuing, with a different model of being a vicar from the normal one. Rather than the all-singing, all-dancing do-it-all-yourself vicar, I model the more general human condition: the struggling survivor.

Chapter Twenty-One

The Darkness Deepens

As my journal entries progress, darkness recurs more frequently. Lack of self-confidence, guilt about my job, guilt about the burdens imposed on people I love, haunt the pages; but then come moments of light:

> On Tuesday morning, I lay in bed, realizing that I needed to forgive myself and let it go... The flagpole of the tower was silhouetted against a clear blue sky, like a thin accusing finger. From right to left an aeroplane passed overhead leaving a brilliant vapour trail over the point. Slowly it spread and sank, forming a white horizontal bar to the vertical black pole. Then at right angles another plane crossed in the sky, laying its vapour trail across the first, to create a shining recumbent plus-sign, which spread and gradually dissolved, as I watched. Clear blue sky was left.

It's as though the disease is an increasingly confining house, prison even, which threatens to become progressively darker as you lose the strength, and then the will, to open the shutters each morning. This is your reality. Gradually you come to believe that your dark enclosure is the real world. There is no more. Just the struggle to survive, to stand, to eat, to clean yourself, to sleep, to breathe. Just the battle with growing dependence and incipient anger at your helplessness. This consumes your waking mind; it invades your dreams. You distract yourself with piped entertainment, so readily on tap, from radio, television and laptop, but however much it is hyped it's like a failing light bulb; returns diminishing each time it's switched on. The walls of the house close in. It's an effort even to open your eyes.

Yet, just occasionally, a wind blows the shutters open and you see some glimpse of the world beyond the walls. Or someone comes and opens them for you, and you are reminded that your now is not the only reality; it's not the whole thing. There is more. Once you walked on the beach at the sea's throbbing edge; once you relished the rain and looked for the rainbow; once you climbed the peaks beside the tumbling, fern-dripping stream. Once you knew that life was good. That's still true. Just because it's dark where you are does not mean there's no light. Even if the shutters were locked and never opened, the sun would still rise and set.

I am sitting in the car on my own at Llangasty, looking across Llangorse Lake, cradled in low-lying hills on the edge of the Brecon Beacons. This is a much-loved place. As a family, we used to stay near Abergavenny at Easter time with friends from Hertfordshire. It was one of our favourite expeditions to come here and walk round the lake's edge as far as we could. Now, Jane is walking the dog on her own. No other cars are here. I am alone. It's an overcast winter's day. The water is steel grey, with the continually shifting pattern of shadow and light, of the wind running over it. A cormorant, flying low and black, skims over the lake's surface. A pair of tufted ducks float across in front of me. A juvenile swan glides past. Through the wind's bluster and the constantly moving bulrushes, as if from a distance, I can hear the subdued chatter of birds and waterfowl and the occasional seagull's cry. Brambles which have still not lost their leaves, even though it's January, weave themselves through the wire fence which stretches out into the water, its posts descending through the flooded lake.

Suddenly the sun breaks through, picking out the colours in the hills running down to the lake and lighting up – what hitherto I've been unable to make out – the many birds on the lake. The clouds break up overhead. To my right, the bracken on the higher hills glows red like embers. At the water's edge the wind-shaken rushes flame gold. There is such beauty – and such longing. In front of me and beside me are stiles, invitations to explore. I know what is on the other side, because I have been there before. However, now I am rooted to my seat by unresponsive muscles. It's no use protesting or raving against my impotence. It's just how it is. I don't like it. Sometimes I sense the rage rising. I wish I could be up and about; I wish I could be walking with Jane; I wish I could stand in the hide along the shoreline and watch the birds through binoculars; I wish ... But really such wishing is futile, that sort of regret a waste of emotion; that anger would be destructive both of myself and of those around me. A wise person in my situation once said that he allowed himself five minutes of self-pity a day and no more. Yes, that's enough.

So my journal is a sort of dialogue between my new limited world and what lies outside. I cannot, with honesty, deny the light-bursts, any more than the dark physical frustrations which run like an ever more insistent ground-bass month by month. There are roses tangled with the briers. I suppose the truth is that roses evolved from briers.

Chapter Twenty-Two

Enigma

I often wonder what to make of all of this. I mean, on the one hand it might be just an experience of accelerated decay. Some people derive a strange excitement from expediting their own mortality. They seem to have a death wish. I'm not one of them. I enjoy the rich tapestry which is life. I derive satisfaction from my work. I love the company of friends and family; yet I don't find solitude lonely. Life is good. I am not in any hurry to die.

Richard Hammond, the *Top Gear* presenter, joked in his cool commentary about the possibility of dying before his 283 mph crash in the jet-propelled 'car' in Yorkshire. The adrenaline rush of travelling so fast made him feel 'so alive'. In retrospect, however, in the studio, it was clear he was grateful merely to be alive, after so close a brush with death. I suspect he is typical of all but a few of those who claim to court their own demise. When it comes to it, they would choose life, not death, every time.

However, I am aware that in the torture chambers of depression, the mind can be so tormented that all light is dark, and death appears preferable to life. That seems to me an unimaginably horrible place to be, far worse than where I am.

O the mind, mind has mountains; cliffs of fall
Frightful, sheer, no-man-fathomed. Hold them cheap
May who ne'er hung there. Nor does long our small
Durance deal with that steep or deep. Here! creep,
Wretch, under a comfort serves in a whirlwind: all
Life death does end and each day dies with sleep.[1]

I know I have not reached that place. I do not look forward to it. I don't know how long my endurance could deal with it. In that sense, my experience is only provisional – but then so must be all our conclusions.

One of my inspirations is my aunt, Susan, now aged 96,[2] who lives in Amesbury. We go to visit her quite often. She is both physically more mobile and mentally more agile than me. Although her eyesight has degenerated, she regularly completes the most difficult cryptic crosswords. During the war she worked for two and a half years at Bletchley Park, where the Enigma code was broken. The hut where she worked, No 6, dealt with the German army and air force signals. She vividly recounts the nights and days spent cracking each day's new code, which was then passed on to Hut No 3, where the messages were decoded and subsequently forwarded straight to Churchill's War Office, or to Montgomery, or wherever. One still senses the excitement of breakthrough.

No one at the moment knows the code to crack MND. And I don't have the code to understand the 'Why?' of it all, either. I have no doubt that one day the pathology and the cure of the disease will be discovered. As to the 'Why?' I guess, like most of the big questions, it will remain a matter of seeing through 'a glass darkly', or puzzling reflections in a very inadequate mirror. But we can, and do, and should, still ask the questions.

The first and most frequently reiterated questions concern the suffering caused by the illness. It's not alone, of course, in being cruel for the patient. There are many diseases which are humiliating and painful, but MND is one of them. I read a vivid description of a man in America lying unable to move or shout for help while ants swarmed up his bed and over his body.[3] By the end, that elusive concept, that universal 'right', quality of life, to all appearances departs completely. The patient is totally dependent on others for everything. He or she has no independent life. They sense they are only a burden and a nuisance. Surely then is the time to allow them to die. And so we come to a raft of connected questions, tied together by a thread of reasonable compassion. Is not euthanasia justified in this case? And is physician-assisted suicide not a legitimate option? And what about living wills made earlier, relieving others of hard choices for the terminally ill? Are there not merciful, humane, exceptions to the absolute sanctity of life and to doctors' duty to preserve life – and is not this one of them? Apparently, the majority of people in the United Kingdom think so. To most of us it seems arrogant and heartless to insist on prolonging another's suffering on a 'mere' matter of principle, when we aren't in their shoes. How dare we?

On 12 May 2006 Lord Joffe introduced the second reading of the Assisted Dying for the Terminally Ill Bill to the UK Parliament's House of Lords. After hours of high-powered debate, which made surprisingly good reading, it was deferred for six months (in effect defeated) by 148 to 100 votes. During the debate, there were religious and non-religious people taking opposite sides, but those I found most powerful spoke from personal experience, such as those in the medical professions. Lord Winston, for example, said:

> Five times in my life I have seen people who are dying who have clearly wanted to die and have expressed that wish repeatedly to me, often over several months. On one occasion, I even filmed that, very controversially, in *The Human Body.* A man called Herbie in Ireland, who suffered from mesothelioma, clearly said to the camera, 'I want to die; I wish somebody could end my life.' Herbie lasted for almost 20 months after that time, and in the last six months of his life he said, 'I am so pleased that I was not taken at my word.' I have seen that four other times with patients.[4]

That month I expressed my reservations about assisted dying in our local newsletter, and a neighbour took me kindly but severely to task for wanting to impose my views (based on religious convictions, to which he said I had a right but which he didn't share) on others. He is an engineer. For him, human beings are sophisticated machines, which when they wear out should be allowed to choose the time of their own shutdown. I could understand the attraction of such freedom of choice. Let me choose when I've had enough. It seems so reasonable; yet it left me uneasy.

Paradoxically, I find something subtly selfish about it. No, I need to rephrase that. For all the genuine compassion that undoubtedly motivates those who argue for assisted suicide, I think there is a streak of selfishness whose existence we need to be honest enough to admit and of whose effects we need to beware. That selfishness comes from a number of directions: the state, carers, the patient himself. Maybe it is only partially selfish, but let's not pretend it is *pure* altruism.

Where does the self-interest lie? From the state's point of view, it is primarily economic. It is true that healthcare absorbs a large proportion of the national budget. It is clearly necessary to put limits on such expenditure. In Britain the National Health Service does not have a bottomless purse, and hard choices have to be made as diagnostic techniques and treatments become ever more expensive. The NHS is funded by taxation, which means, ultimately, by the electorate. No political party wants to include increasing taxation in its manifesto; it's a recipe for losing an election. So the pressure to make cuts in (or at least to restrict) healthcare expenditure, without appearing to do so, is strong. The temptation is to go for a soft target, and those who are dying anyway are just that. So are those who are perceived to have a poor quality of life, such as the physically or mentally handicapped. Prolonging life – especially life requiring constant care – is obviously more expensive than shortening it. Palliative care does not come cheap. To find a politically and fiscally acceptable alternative would come as a great relief to governments. Perhaps if they wait long enough and fail to give a strong lead, public opinion will become sufficiently irresistible and our former ethical scruples will have been washed away. What is sinister is the spin which gives a compassionate face to a utilitarian motivation.

With carers, it is rather more personal and complex. There's a difference between professional carers – those whose job it is to care – and wives, husbands, children or whoever with a dependent relative, amateurs in the literal sense – those who do it from love. For them, it is impossible to disentangle the mass of emotions involved. Their lives are devoted to the care of their loved one. Of course they would not have it any other way. Yet, for all the commitment of both amateurs and professionals, there is immense sadness at seeing the wreckage of a human being sinking inexorably beneath the waves. For one thing, it is a painfully vivid reminder of their own mortality: a living *memento mori.* But there is also real personal pain in the act of caring itself. In my experience the most harrowing bereavement is that of a mother for her child: it is the cruel triumph of the unnatural (premature death) over the natural (maternal love). Almost as harrowing, however, is the helpless witnessing of a loved one's suffering. Even the veiled threat of it is recognized as the most potent weapon of torture ('We know where your family are...'). But for it to go on in reality, day after day, month after month, perhaps for years, is too much to bear. No wonder that often, in the end, the amateur hands over to the professional, with varying degrees of reluctance and relief and, of course, guilt. The patient is placed in residential care 'for their own good'. That is probably and usually true, but there is also – it would be naïve to deny – an element of self-interest in such decisions. The carers feel they can't cope any longer; *their* quality of life is zilch; *their* pain has become unbearable. How much of the 'mercy', we might ask, in mercy-killing is for the carer and how much for the patient?

But how on earth can a patient's desire to die with 'dignity' be disfigured with the tag 'selfish'? (By the way, I find 'dignity' a weasel word in this context, as if receiving a lethal dose is in some way more 'dignified' than suffering to the bitter end, whether with stoical acceptance or querulous complaining.) Primarily, I feel, the answer lies in what it demands of the carers. It is saying to them: 'I want you to put *my* wishes first. You may want to cling on to hope. You may treasure the time spent with me, but I've had enough of everything: of the pain, of the struggle, of life, of you.' It demands probably, too, that they take the decision to pull the plug, to end your life – and the sting is that, even if the decision was yours, not all the responsibility for that goes with you into the grave. The carers survive, as an accessory to the act.

And they are not alone. The professional carers are inevitably involved. For doctors and nurses there's a double bind: denying their vocation to save life and compromising their standing as healers. 'For me,' the patient says, 'I want you to break your normal rule of saving life. End mine, because it's not worth living.' Although I personally hate it when I see the wishes of 'clients' in nursing homes being cavalierly ignored, the principle at stake is more a matter of respect for another human being than the violation of a right. The staff are simply transgressing the universal obligation of compassion. Conversely, however, there is almost an arrogance in demanding one's 'rights' or wishes at the expense of other people's needs or integrity. And there's no denying that a dying wish is an exercise of considerable power. I can understand why the continually demanding complainer in a residential home might be discreetly sedated, though I don't think it's justified. Yet to require or allow doctors to administer lethal injections would be to undermine their integrity and position of trust. An ambivalence would enter the doctor–patient relationship. Normally physicians would do all they could to prolong life, but occasionally they might cut it short. Whether you are asking doctors to make the decision to terminate life or merely to carry it out, that is an intolerable reversal of their whole *raison d'être.* I would rather allow them to carry out their calling of care, healing and relief of pain than to make an exception for me. The hospice movement has proved that dying need not be undignified. One can go gentle, but not easily, into the good night.

Notes

[1] From Gerard Manley Hopkins, 'No worst, there is none'.

[2] Susan Wenham died on 21st February 2009, aged 97.

[3] Joni Eareckson Tada and Steven Estes, *When God weeps* (Zondervan, 1997).

[4] *Hansard,* House of Lords, 12 May 2006.

Chapter Twenty-Three

What Price Life?

The questions surround the central theme of the value of a particular human life. Is there some calculus by which we can grade its value, such as productivity x employable years, or intelligence x diligence, or wealth x fame? Is a wage-earner worth more than an unemployed mother? In May 2005 I read that the research team at Newcastle upon Tyne which had produced Dolly the cloned sheep announced that they had successfully produced a human embryo by cell nuclear transfer (as used for Dolly). This was therapeutic cloning for research purposes and was held out as a great hope for research into such diseases as Parkinson's and MND. Baroness Warnock wrote persuasively to counter any moral objections. She concluded that they were outweighed by 'our human duty to pursue, in the spirit of both compassion and understanding, the lead that the Newcastle team has given us. In my view they are greatly to be congratulated for having made a start.'[1]

There was one part of her article which provoked me to write to the trade journal concerned:

> Sir,
>
> With no other qualification than being a potential client myself, may I comment on the contributions of your two eminent ethicists (May 27)? I

was struck by Baroness Warnock's assertion that medical research is 'directed to no other goal than to remedy the ills that tend to make them (human lives) less valuable to those who are living them', not so much for its optimism about the disinterested nature of corporate business, as for its concept of *value.*

I imagine my untreatable degenerative condition is the sort of 'ill' she is referring to. Since contracting it, I have not found my life less valuable: less independent, less predictable, certainly; more frustrating, more restricted, painfully so. But I share this with my elderly neighbours, my disabled colleague, the children of our special needs' schools, others facing terminal illness, and with countless more. Oddly my experience is that life has become more focused and even fulfilled, and, best of all, I've found myself to be valued not for what I can do (which is diminishing) but for who I am – which is embarrassingly but liberatingly humbling. I believe from God it's called grace; from human beings it's love. It's worth being on the receiving end.

I don't know what Baroness Warnock's measure of value is. However, I suspect the question of what makes human lives valuable is one issue at the heart of our moral confusion. Is it how useful, how capable, how 'normal', how pain-free, or how viable they are or even how they are valued by the individual or the rest of society? Or do they have an intrinsic inalienable value which, acknowledged or not, derives from their God-given origin?

Don't get me wrong. To question the implication that illness somehow makes lives affected less valuable is *not* to question the need for cutting-edge research into effective therapies. But Dr Watts is right to point out the dilemma, for patients, created by research on embryos. Should it become possible to offer people like me a cure as a result of cloning, we would face the prospect of our prolonged survival (which is all that 'cures' are, for everyone) at the expense of the creation and destruction of numerous human embryos – too hard a choice for either the patient or their family. No doubt treatment would not be offered in such terms (and one might ask why), but that would not alter the fact of the matter, nor the media-informed universal knowledge of the fact.

I trust that I won't be faced with that choice. I trust that I will see a God-given remedy for intractable conditions, such as mine. Above all, I trust that I will not lose Job's conviction, 'The Lord gave; the Lord has taken away. Blessed be the name of the Lord', because that way lies sanity and even peace.

Not surprisingly, Baroness Warnock won the argument and I lost! Two years later, the UK government, after heavy lobbying from researchers, published a parliamentary Bill to lift the ban on producing hybrid human–animal embryos for medical research. To my untutored ear the very idea of such hybrids sounds bizarre, and creating even the very first seeds of life with intention of destroying them seems perverse. But I know that others with MND are hopeful that it will prove a step on the road to discovering causes and cures, even if many years ahead. The admirable MND Association said, 'Future research into MND will rely upon the technology developed to create human–animal embryos, as a source of stem cells.' The Association's research manager, Dr Belinda Cupid, was delighted. 'We hope that progress in this area will not be further delayed and that MND researchers can now work towards the Association's vision of a world free of MND.'[2] On 19th May 2008, the bill was debated in the House of Commons and a ban on hybrids was defeated by a majority of 160.

It is an irony that in our anxiety to prolong our lives we hold life itself cheap. This contradiction makes for a precarious endeavour. We may see a world free of MND. I believe we shall. But we will never make a world free of death. What matters even more is that we place an infinite value on human life. So we cannot afford to abuse that life, especially when it is vulnerable. I suppose the debate is what constitutes human life and when it begins.

Yet I believe my main point will always remain true. When we lose everything, all is not lost, in particular our selves. As one fictional mother observed when her son had lost everything he had worked and she had hoped for: '...all worldly mortification sank to nothing before the consciousness of the great blessing that he himself by his simple existence was to her.'[3] In the unprecedented prosperity of the West in the twenty-first century, we risk undervaluing mere existence.

Notes

[1] *Church of England Newspaper,* 27 May 2005.

[2] Press statement, 17 May 2007.

[3] Mrs Thornton, in Elizabeth Gaskell, *North and South* (Wordsworth Editions, 2002), p.393.

Chapter Twenty-Four

But What If...?

I wake up in the night, and Jane is missing. She's not there beside me. I strain to hear any sound of movement. Where is she? Is she in the house? Has she fallen in the bathroom and hit her head? How could I reach her? I can't even get out of bed without her. My imagination slips the leash. Cold fear begins to rise. I'm helpless. And then I hear the toilet flush, the bedroom door opens and Jane climbs back into bed. But for once I lie there, awake, contemplating: 'What if she wasn't around? What if she had an accident or was ill? Where would that leave me?'

Without Jane I would long ago have had to give up work. I'd have lost mobility. Jane was able to tell me when I was no longer safe on the road, in her opinion, and she was willing to drive me to all my engagements from early morning to late evening. I'd have perhaps graduated to driving an adapted car, assuming I'd not lost control before, but some time ago even that would have been no use, as I wouldn't have been able to get into or out of it.

Shopping would be impossible, except of course by internet. Holidays would be out of the question, making my life much duller – no weeks away in Dorset, Wales or Lancashire. My social life would shrink: no weddings, or meals out. The daily essentials are beyond me on my own, from getting up to going to bed. I can't get dressed and undressed, showered and dried. I can't cook myself a meal, or wash up afterwards. Tidying up is a lengthy, monumental effort, and, as my reach is so limited, remains partial at best. It would not be long before I was smelly, unkempt and undernourished, surrounded by squalor. If I fell, I'd have to stay where I landed, with any injuries, until someone happened by, unless I had remembered to put my mobile in a pocket to ring 999. Actually it wouldn't be long before I was lingeringly dying. I know that our family would step in, but there's no escaping how dependent on someone else I really am.

I wonder how I would cope with carers coming in three times a day – the last resort before being institutionalized. I can't imagine exposing so much of my intimate life to strangers. Yet I know many people do, because they have no choice. I suppose it's like being in hospital in your own home, with long periods of isolation between visits. But even that must be preferable to being indefinitely confined to a nursing home, mustn't it? Sometimes at night we can hear the haunting repetitive shouts from the home behind the hedge bordering our garden: 'Nurse ... Nurse ... Nurse ... Nurse...' You never know how silence is restored, whether by a reassuring word, or a sedative, or some other remedy. But the forlornness hangs in the air.

Nevertheless, I recall Greta, the caretaker from the church school in Wantage, who had MND and whose husband, Eric, had senile dementia. The two of them were admitted to our local nursing home, since there was no way that she could care for him any more at home. With silvery grey hair and plastic-rimmed spectacles, she had a sweet nature and would sit with Eric even when he was beyond communicating with her. Occasionally, though, he would join her for communion. And he came to the party which was put on in the village hall for her last birthday. We could do nothing but watch as the disease quite quickly deprived her muscles of strength. The MND Association provided her with a panoply of aids, which she enjoyed demonstrating when we visited. Soon Greta was unable to come into the lounge; she was confined to her bed, with remote controls for lights and radio. She had frightening bouts of breathlessness at nights, but although she told me about them I never heard her complain. She died, I believe, from a chest infection. She was a brave little lady. She made the best of what she had. It doesn't have to be defeat. She was apprehensive about the road, but I don't think she was afraid of where death led to.

Round and round go the night thoughts on the 'What if?' carousel. In the end I resort to my dismount tactics: devices to stop the circulating thoughts. First I try the mental maths tack: I look at the alarm clock. Its red LCD figures read 2:47. The question is: ignoring the colon, is that a prime number? I experiment with the possible factors. Yes. I look again: 2:50. How many ways can that be divided? Too easy. So I turn over and reach up to the radio. I switch on the BBC World Service, turn it down so that it doesn't disturb Jane and start to listen. The trick is setting the right volume, audible but not intrusive. This is sure-fire. The same news comes round every half-hour, and in between are some programmes which are just interesting enough to engage but not hold my attention. If there's cricket from the other side of the world (Five Live Sports Extra), that's normally even better, because nothing much happens that, as an Englishman, one wants to hear. When my own roundabout has slowed to a stop and I'm dozing, I usually manage to reach and switch it off. And peace is restored.

The answer to the question, 'But what if my circumstances were different?' is, it would leave me in the same place as many others, and then perhaps I might not be so resistant to assisted suicide, or ambivalent about stem-cell research. I guess I might be desperate to be anywhere except where I was. I don't want to be complacent in my own situation. It is of course futile and illegitimate to speculate on what might have been. I suppose my intention is to admit how lucky I am, and therefore how hard it is for others. I cannot imagine it yet. As well, I find myself among the ardent admirers of 'the carers'. Even when they receive an allowance, whatever it is, they are worth more, but what's most extraordinary – and most right – is that the majority do it for nothing but love. As their number increases, so society's support for them needs to grow, not so much in monetary terms, but in real and tangible honour for what they do. It is costly, but still, in my book, caring to the end of life is a better way than caring enough to end life.

Chapter Twenty-Five

The Consolation of Religion

You could be forgiven for thinking from the letter I wrote to the paper that I take refuge in the religious dogmas that are my stock in trade. Although the truths which I believe are foundational to me, they do not, I find, provide a balm to soften the acuteness of pain. Convictions do not lessen hunger pangs. Toothache is not eased by faith. Depression is not charmed away. I'm not immunized against nighttime fears.

The eponymous hero of the ancient cross between an epic and a drama, Job, is a devout and thoroughly good man. However, when disaster strikes in appalling totality, neither his own faith nor the extensive religious platitudes of his four comforters succeed in mitigating his suffering; if anything, they exacerbate his pain and frustration. Quite early on in my illness, a friend of many years' standing who is a psychologist took the trouble to make me face reality. 'You are in a bereavement situation, Michael. And so is your family and the church family. You need to allow them to grieve. You must not let your MND be a taboo subject.' She was, of course, quite right in every respect. In my determination to carry on as normally as possible, I was in danger of forcing denial on others as well as myself – a futile and toxic waste of time.

Nicola wisely helped me to recognize my escalating loss. Whether I feel miserable or not – and most of the time I don't – I am in a state of bereavement. I have lost much of my life. C.S. Lewis was probably the greatest defender of Christian faith in the twentieth century. When his wife, Joy Gresham, died after a prolonged and painful fight with cancer, he kept a record of his thoughts. They were later published (at first using the pen name N.W. Clerk) under the title of *A Grief Observed.* It is as honest an account of grief from the inside as I know. At one point he writes:

> Talk to me about the truth of religion and I'll listen gladly. Talk to me about the duty of religion and I'll listen submissively. But don't come talking to me about the consolations of religion or I shall suspect that you don't understand.[1]

That last sentence has resonated with me ever since I first read it.

One evening we were talking about the common notion that religious belief is a crutch. 'That's nonsense,' said our friend. She wasn't old. She had been married twice. I'd taken one of the services. She'd been divorced twice. She had had major heart surgery. You could often hear the artificial valve clicking away inside her. 'It's not true. It's simply that when everything else has been taken away, there's just you – and God. That's the moment of truth. You decide. It's not a crutch.' Faith hadn't made her life any easier.

Don't come talking to me about the consolations of religion. Not that my faith leaves me cold or without resource – far from it – but it raises more painful questions than it provides answers. I would not advocate it as a panacea for pain. There may be some evidence that it aids the healing process, but it doesn't reduce the hurting a jot. Instead, the person with faith in a divine Creator is forced to ask a lot of 'Why?' questions which need never bother an atheist. Why is suffering such a widespread phenomenon in the work of a good God? Why has it affected me (or a member of my family) particularly acutely? Is there intention behind pain, or is it mere accident? How do I square this with what I used to believe about a God who loves me? If God is all-powerful and if he's all-loving, why does he not *do* something? Why do children, the innocent, suffer? These are hard questions which humans have been asking, I suspect, from the time they first began reflecting. So, ironically, there's potential for a double downward spiral, of both physical weakness and undermined faith, in a chronic disease, which in normal circumstances you would be able to steer around. However, now, you cannot avoid wondering, and of course you have the time to dwell on your thoughts, as you sit in your chair waiting to be helped to eat, or as you find yourself increasingly embarrassing.

There's potential for dark despair as to your value and attractiveness. When questions arise concerning your God's compassion, you are tempted to wonder whether it is compassion or pity that you read in people's eyes and actions. Am I becoming merely an object of pity? Is that all that's left to me?

Religion can also be a breeding ground for guilt, of course, with its moral imperatives, such as the Ten Commandments and the even more stringent teachings of Jesus, and consequences of eternal reward and punishment. Lurking at the threshold of consciousness, therefore, crouches the dark accuser, whispering, 'You deserve this. This is all your fault. You've brought this on yourself and your family.' And you're invited to enter a cycle of introspection and cancerous self-blame. It's a half-baked sort of religion which thinks like this, but it's reinforced by well-meant comments such as 'I can't understand why it should happen to you,' or 'What have they done to deserve all that?' These are well-meant, because they are supposed to exonerate the sufferer, but at the same time they reinforce the widely held, superstitious belief that suffering is an individually deserved punishment. As Rogers and Hammerstein might have put it: 'so somewhere in my youth or childhood, I must have done something bad.' (The converse is equally absurd, I'm afraid.) And so there is the danger that you subconsciously buy in to that mindset.

I have to admit that there is in what I would call true religion a consciousness of 'sin', which often brings with it undesirable consequences, or penalties. These consequences, however, are inherent in the action, rather than arbitrarily imposed. To give a simplistic example, a child running across a busy road without looking risks the inherent consequence of being hit by a car. He also runs a risk of the arbitrary but not unreasonable pain of being smacked by an anxious parent. It seems to me that God is in the business of inherent rather than arbitrary consequences. He doesn't smack us (or strike us with thunderbolts) when we're naughty, but he does allow our actions to have consequences. He permits us that dignity. However, he does more than that. Much of the time, he lets us know, whether by research or revelation, 'This is caused by that.' We can work out that atom bombs and cigarettes result in cancers. Similarly, my MND may have a cause, unknown to me and to doctors at present, arising from some circumstance in my life. Some day an avoidable environmental or lifestyle factor may be identified. Nevertheless, there is no evidence to support the view that God inflicts individuals with disease as a form of retribution, and some to the contrary – in my view at least.

Note

[1] C.S. Lewis, *A Grief Observed* (Faber, 1966), p.23.

Chapter Twenty-Six

Healing

One puzzling phenomenon to me, brought up and educated within the Western scientific tradition, is the fact of medically unexplained recovery from 'untreatable' conditions. In some circles these are claimed as miracles; in some they are written off as fabrication; and sometimes judgment is reserved. They are regarded as 'unexplained' recoveries or remissions. Personally, I am tempted to sit on the fence and say that all three may occur. However, I cannot honestly say I'm comfortable or satisfied with that position, if it means maintaining an open mind in every case. The problem with a permanently open mind is that it never closes on a conclusion. Of course, minds can be prematurely closed. If you have prejudged the issue of a supernatural dimension to life and written it off as impossible, then you won't entertain the 'miracle' option. But I have seen enough extraordinary recoveries – and heard of more from witnesses I judge to be reliable – to lead me to the conclusion that there are more things in heaven and earth than our philosophy has dreamed of.

I have met someone healed of inoperable cancer after being prayed for, and someone cured of multiple sclerosis after praying. I've seen people walking – even leaping – having been crippled with arthritis.

Not long ago, a week after a service in which we prayed for her healing, Ness, a friend of ours, sent us an email. She had

> a hearing problem which was investigated a year ago, and was prayed for to ask that it was nothing serious like a tumour which I was to attend an MRI scan for. It wasn't serious, but as a result of this investigation I was told I had lost 30–40% hearing in my left ear, probably 3 years ago when Oliver was born. I was told this was due to a viral infection, which I remember I had at the time, and that nothing could be done because it was nerve damage. I have had to live for the last three years with this hearing problem. During the normal course of the day this is not too troublesome because my right ear has perfect hearing and compensates for the loss in the left. It is more of a bother at night if I am lying on my good ear as I find it hard to hear properly without sound becoming quite muffled. John always says I had started to use this to my advantage by not hearing the children or the alarm clock of a morning!

The next few days after the prayer were quite eventful.

> The following Wednesday I awoke as usual and was lying on my good ear and could hear Oliver up and about. I asked John, 'Why is Oliver shouting?' John replied that he wasn't shouting – how odd I thought – I sat up and lay back down

> several times to find to my amazement that there seemed to be no difference between my hearing in my left and right ear. We tried several more 'tests' and true enough my hearing was as good as my right ear. This has continued to be the case and if anything sounds are very acute at the moment, and I am forever asking John to turn the TV down or not to talk so loud!

Not so dramatic, perhaps, as witnessing a withered arm grow to normal, as I heard described from South Africa, or seeing whitened blind eyes return to their natural colour and perfect sight (in Mozambique), or a wheelchair-bound woman stand up and dispense with her chair for good (in England), but just as inexplicable – except for their only common denominator being the element of prayer. I have to confess that personally I have seen more people die who have been prayed for. And, of course, I have seen many more people cured of disease by conventional medicine and surgery, although all of these have died or will die in the end. But at least I cannot honestly dismiss the miraculous.

This leads me to another painful puzzle of faith. Why haven't I received a miracle? (I use 'miracle' as a shorthand for – depending on your viewpoint – an unexplained recovery by chance, or from so far not understood causes, or from God's intervention in response to prayer.) If you believe that miracles can and do happen, then there's that possibility. I have been told that I have a right to be healed, just as long as I have sufficient faith: a sort of religious variant of mind over matter. I went to one massive 'healing' rally based on this philosophy, where some people *were* remarkably cured, but I shan't forget sitting behind one young man in a wheelchair desperately trying to believe he was healed and still unable to stand, nor the weary families wheeling their children back to their Motability vehicles, out of the arena into the night. They had come in good faith; they left disappointed, because of the hype. However, I don't believe in a slot-machine God: 'You pays your money; you gets your wish.' I have been prayed for many times: in person, I mean. I understand that people pray for me every day, on their own. I remain ill. Yet I like being prayed for. For one thing, I always feel better afterwards! My opinion is that this is more than psychological, though it would be none the worse for that; I sense that through prayer there is always an encounter with God, who, as the children's book puts it, is not tame, but who *is* love.

Chapter Twenty-Seven

The Final Question

If it is true that God is love, then disease and disaster raise a towering dark question mark over our concept of love, and for me, as a Christian, over my pictures of a God who loves. Perhaps this has become so ingrained in my subconscious that it stubbornly resists repeated attempts at erasing it. However, thus far in my illness, my conclusion has been that in talking about the love behind existence we are dealing with something far deeper, more severe and more mysterious than anything we bargained for. This seems to be borne out by the event at the centre of Christianity. I don't use worry beads or prayer beads for that matter, but the rosary, the Catholic version, provides for me a visual image of the mystery. Strung together are the fifty beads, spheres providing no point of rest or reference. As fingers wander over them, so minds wrestle over the hard questions of existence and find no resolution. It seems a never-ending cycle. But uniquely, in the rosary, in the middle is the awkward and ugly shape of the crucifix: a gallows and an agonized dying figure. Why is it there? Somehow, it seems, it is the key to the unresolved cycle – God transfixed in human pain. That, if anything, is severe. It is certainly a mystery. It provides no neat answers to the worry beads.

At Christmas 2003, I saw a card picturing the stable at Bethlehem which struck me as somewhat sentimental; so I wrote:

Jesus, the amazing thing is that you ever came out of *that* stable – electrically lit, comfortably air-conditioned, conveniently spacious it looks ... out into the unremitting heat of the Middle Eastern day – occupied, violent, diseased, divided; out into the relentless dark of nights, freezing strongholds of fear, where in the end you would face weakness, pain and the enemy's final weapon, administered with merciless savagery. You knew what was coming, even before this moment; you knew what lay in store with perfect clarity when you made your decision. You knew what lay ahead, every step you took, every roadside execution you passed, every grief-prostrated family you met, every God-forsaken hostage of satan, whose desperation threw them at your feet.

You knew it was all coming to you – and more. No wonder you set your face like flint. No wonder you begged to be let off. No wonder you cried. No wonder you sweated terror-blood. The wonder is that you ever left that place of light. The wonder is that you didn't duck out. The wonder is that you didn't call back that army of angels to give you a pain-free exit strategy. The wonder is that you let the nails hold up your blood-draining, breath-gulping,

> convulsing body through and beyond endurance.
>
> Why? The wonder is you died so soon, so young. Only the naïve imagine the resurrection made it easier. So why? Tell me, why you did it. Why? I need to know.

But does believing in life after death not make it easier? That's part of the religious deal, isn't it? People talk about 'pie in the sky when you die' as a compensation for a raw deal in life. Even if it reflected the truth, it actually doesn't address or alleviate the rawness of life. Nice ideas don't anaesthetize sustained pain. Pain can be a long dark tunnel with no end in sight, when walking is a hopeless effort of the will. Or it can be blindingly acute, like needles of inescapable sunlight burning your retinas. Or it can be sheer weariness, when your whole system screams, or whimpers, 'Enough! I've had enough!' Positive thinking is powerless then. That's when it is irrelevant to talk about the consolation of religion.

I'm not saying that belief in life after death is irrelevant, or unimportant, but simply that it doesn't impact at the point of pain. Its particular impact is on life itself. It means that my actions do not end with my death, for me any more than for those who survive me. For better or worse, they matter, and continue to matter. It gives existence an eternal weight of significance. At the same time it suggests a perspective beyond our limited horizons.

The walker disappears into the mist. It tells me I do not see the whole picture. My attempts to make sense of what I experience are based on essentially inadequate data. 'Now we see in a glass darkly...'

'...but then face to face.' That's what Louise, my friend, anticipates. There is a reality more real than ours. Our living will be seen to have been the dream.

> There is no growing old in the age to come. Those of us who struggled on earth with disability, disease or deformity enjoy freedom from the bondage to decay. No more wasted muscles, heart disease, cancer, arthritic joints or wheezy chests. There is no more death, no mourning, no crying, no pain!
>
> Can you even imagine?
>
> The eyes of the blind are opened and the ears of the deaf unstopped. The lame leap like the deer, and the mute tongue shouts for joy!
>
> And in heaven I do not need to find alternatives to dancing. Here, I have the REAL THING. When I dance, my feet twist to the hip hop beat in worship and I twirl on my tiptoe to the sound of a heavenly symphony!
>
> The age to come is full of creativity – art, poetry, song, dancing, music for every taste, science, inventing, creating, thinking, talking, listening, praising. For the first time ever we are truly equipped to walk in the spirit.

> Those of us who hungered to be filled more fully with the Spirit of God, are filled to overflowing. Our emotions are at peace and there are waves of joy washing over us.
>
> Even the rains are glorious. And the trees of the fields clap their hands!
>
> And when I spend time in my room – the room in my Father's house already prepared for me, I relax in worship in the light of the dawn.
>
> Those who struggled on earth to find a true home, at last have a real sense of belonging, a real sense of home, a deep sense of rest – a home where we can eat good food, where there are healing oils and wine and where we are *truly* satisfied.
>
> The dream is ended. THIS is the morning![1]

Of course, this is an optimistic vision, predicated on the belief in a good God at the heart of existence, and there is no denying that that belief provides a powerful and deeper counterpoint to the frustrations of increased weakness and dependency. However, it is not a new vision, but one that has its roots in prophetic seeings over thousands of years. It has been a powerful source of hope, but not pain relief, to races and individuals under the cosh ever since. 'Hope is the conviction that all we live for, happiness and sorrow, victory and defeat, will be found to have some sense' (Timothy Radcliffe OP).[2] That's my conviction too.

Notes

[1] From 'Heaven Vision', written by Louise Halling in 2005.

[2] Quoted by Anthony Sutch on *Today,* BBC Radio 4, 20 June 2007.

Chapter Twenty-Eight

In the Meantime

Nevertheless, if that's the morning, the evening continues to close in. So it's back to the present time. That is then; but this is now. It has been some months since I began writing, and although I'm told how well I'm doing I can detect the cracks continuing to spread and to deepen.

For 'walking' any distance I use an electric wheelchair from home, or if we are away, a manual one. No longer do I insist on walking with a stick, leaning on Jane's arm. Walking a hundred yards is an achievement, and I've had enough by the end. I enjoy using my wheelchair, not least because it once belonged to my neighbour, Jock Hamilton-Baillie, the former Colditz prisoner and brigadier-general. It was passed on to me by his son and refurbished by courtesy of the NHS. It allows me to get out and talk to people without the constant anxiety of losing my balance. I can still – and do – physically walk around the house with my Rollator, wanting to maintain mobility as long as possible. But my knees rub together and my feet step on each other. So I stumble and have the occasional fall. I'm fortunate to have had Jane and Bryan on hand to pick me up! Coming down the stairs, my legs may go into spasm, and I have to pause, shifting my balance, until the shaking stops.

The NHS went through a transformation in Oxford with the closure of the Infirmary, where my consultations were based, and the opening of the state-of-the-art West Wing at the John Radcliffe Hospital. It is an impressive piece of modern design, but the planners failed to anticipate the perils for the elderly visually impaired of having the eye department at the top of some escalators. At least the casualty department is not far away. It was some time before I got to see it. The month of my annual appointment came and went. I heard nothing. Rumour had it that staff had been told to cut their patient lists by 10 per cent to save money. So routine appointments had been put on hold for six months. 'Am I one of those, or was my file lost in the move?' I wondered darkly, and I fondly remembered a year previously, when I had rung a consultant and found myself talking not to a secretary but to the man himself, who immediately arranged for a home visit from the mobility scientist.

In the end I did hear from the West Wing. There had been a cancellation. Could I go in? It was a slightly eerie experience: no hunting for on-street parking, but parking round and beneath the multi-storey building – at a price. None of the old-world corridors and crowded waiting rooms of the Infirmary; instead lifts, glass and airy consulting rooms – utilitarian, and somewhat impersonal, until we reached the familiar figure of Dr Donaghy, who was immediately engaged. Here at least, I'm still treated as a person, not a case, or even a patient. He seems laid back, but his observation is acute. He does not take long to assess me, and we then talk about the options for the future. He is happy to allow me my autonomy, but repeats that he's available whenever I feel I need to consult him. I appreciate that. So, reassured and pencilled in for next year, we descend in the lift, pay the parking fee and head for the rush-hour traffic on the ring road.

At home, we've had the bath taken out and replaced with a shower cubicle in which I can sit down. It makes the experience of showering a great deal more pleasurable, and, although entering and exiting is a far from simple manoeuvre, it is considerably safer than having to vault over the side of the bath. In point of fact, vaulting is hardly a good description of the stage I had reached; it was more a teetering balancing act with stiffly uncooperative limbs, putting both Jane, propping and catching me, and myself in increasing peril of landing in a heap on one side of the bath or the other. My employers and landlords, Oxford Diocese, were very willing to make the change. The only down side is for the rest of the family, including the dog, who are now denied a bath.

Eating is even slower now. It's becoming harder to grip the cutlery, and courting disaster to talk and eat. So, silently and painstakingly, I cut up my food and carefully chew it, fishing errant bits out from behind my teeth. My brain needs to process what's on the menu, and so I tend not to mix mouthfuls – always assuming I can persuade the food to stay on the fork between the plate and my mouth. I'll have the pizza first, then the peas, and finally – having taken long enough for it to cool down – the baked potato.

I feel I have reverted to the last schoolboy in the Nissen-hut dining hall of my childhood... It's bread-and-butter pudding, my least favourite dessert. Everyone else has finished, and they're all waiting for me. The sadistic French teacher, with his protruding belly and black moustache, stands over me. 'We're all waiting for you, Wenham,' he hisses loudly. Every half-spoonful makes my gorge rise. Eventually, he dismisses the rest. 'Not you, Wenham!' he snarls. 'You are going nowhere until that plate's clean.' Outside, the sun is shining. There's shouting and laughter from the playground. 'I'm waiting,' Hitler breathes darkly down my neck. I force myself to swallow another mouthful, hide the rest under my spoon, and put my hand up. 'Sir, I've finished. Can I go now, please?' He stalks over, looks at my plate and lifts the spoon. I think I'm going to be sick. 'Eat it, boy!' I put the final dollop of cold congealed school bread and margarine and egg-powder pudding in my mouth, hoping to make a run to the toilet and spit it out. 'Swallow it.' I try to hold it under my tongue and do a pretend gulp. But he's merciless. 'Open your mouth.' He inspects. 'Swallow!' It goes, and so do I. But the bell is ringing. Lunch-time is over, and last lesson is French.

The horror of being last, of keeping the others waiting, has deep roots. I have no personal Hitlers now; in fact, quite the opposite. My companions will quite happily sit it out while I, somewhat messily and noisily, finish each course. It's just that buried shadow rearing its moustachioed head. But it can't be *too* bad, as my waist size has increased. I'm far from wasting away.

My increasing waistline may also be a product of deteriorating muscles. I guess I don't even have a one-pack. It's not a localized problem. Despite the use of elephant feet, getting up from chairs has become more and more difficult, especially in the evenings. (Elephant feet are conical devices to put under chair or bed legs to give them three or more inches of extra height – which of course makes standing up easier, as you are that much nearer the vertical.) Techniques which once worked are no longer so effective, as muscles weaken, bit by bit, in legs and arms. This is accentuated when we go on holiday and stay in an unfamiliar place. Then I have to learn new tricks for unfamiliar seats, beds, toilets, washing and just getting around. Quite often I tweak a muscle repeatedly, a nuisance which can assume unwarranted proportions, and then Jane has to put up with my thespian sighs and grimaces. Nevertheless, for me holidays are worth it as an antidote to the closing-in which the disease brings and as a recharging of physical and mental energy. It doesn't take many weeks of work before rising from my highest chair and dragging myself with leaden feet up the stairs at the end of the day seems the final straw. It would be easier just to remain there and wait for the morning to come.

Chapter Twenty-Nine

The Shape of Things to Come?

Then it gets worse.

'Have you passed your test for that?' I'm driving through the churchyard in my electric wheelchair. It's the standard quip, but it still amuses Les, the jovial gravedigger. George, the local undertaker, joins in: 'He's faster than Lewis Hamilton on that thing, aren't you, Michael?' They're standing in the middle of graves, finding the reserved plot for a burial after the weekend. They're always up for a laugh, and on this sunny autumnal day they're in an especially jocular mood. As I drive away, bumping over the hazardous tree-root ridges on the path, George has his parting shot: 'You just go carefully on that machine...' Laughing, I go on my way down through the village to assembly at the local primary school.

It's a shame that I don't speak well enough to take assemblies any more. I used to enjoy that, and being active in the school. I suppose it was a nostalgic throwback to my teaching days. Quite early on in my MND, I felt sufficiently embarrassed to stop coming to school at all, once I couldn't get there under my own steam. It was the advent of the wheelchair that gave me sufficient independence to return, though this time as a silent, benevolent spectator from the back of the hall. The children have become used to seeing me there, but only the bravest dare smile in the solemnity of the occasion. Marshalled like troops on parade, they sit and stand in straight and silent rows. As they file out by me, I feel a bit like the Queen at a march past: 'Eyes right!' The teachers are a friendly lot, but I don't know them so well now. Occasionally I join them for a quick cup of coffee in the staff room after assembly, but today someone's coming to see me at 11.15, and I need to get back.

The head teacher sees me out. I've just handed over a cheque; so she gives me a particularly friendly goodbye. As usual, I do a wide sweep to the right to round the gatepost and keep on the pavement. However, I miscalculate. My speed is too fast, my reactions too slow, and the right front wheel goes over the kerb. Half the wheelchair follows and tips over, taking me with it. The wheelchair is relatively undamaged, but that's thanks to my shoulder which has taken the full force of the impact. I lie there on the High Street, with a sidelong view across to the Business Centre, wondering what will happen next. I can't shout; I can't move; I can't reach my mobile in my pocket. There seems to be no one in sight. I don't know whether to hope for a car to come or not. My arm is grazed, but I'm not aware of other injuries. It's just that I can't move. The seconds stretch into minutes, it seems. I'm sure it's not that long before an elderly gentleman comes from the Co-op, walking on the other side of the road. I assume he summons help, as he, together with a man in painter's overalls and someone in a business suit, come across to sort me out.

I hear a van swing round the bend, but it's not going fast and pulls up opposite. I am not articulate enough to explain what's wrong with me, but my rescuers can see enough. They right the wheelchair, and manhandle me back into it. The only time it hurts is when my right armpit is used as a lifting point. The wheelchair's not working, and the clutch is engaged, which makes moving it off the road a matter of brute strength. Once out of harm's way, someone reconnects the battery and we have power, and they're able to move me back into the school's forecourt. That's when the shock sets in.

By now, a teaching assistant has seen me and summoned help from the staff room. Janet, the teacher, who knows me well, telephones Jane on my mobile. The scarlet first-aid blanket appears and is wrapped over me. I gather it contrasts well with my putty grey colour. I feel that I'm passing out. Dimly I wonder whether I'll be sick. In time it passes, and the familiar sound of our car's diesel engine comes round the corner. Jane soon realizes, however, that there's no way I can get into it or be lifted in. We decide to make for home, Jane pushing the heavy wheelchair with me on board. On the uphill section we engage the motor, and I find I can control it with my right fingers. I feel slightly absurd as, covered in my bright red blanket, I pass members of my congregation coming from a service. I vainly try to look normal.

It's good to get home, but as I go into shock again, it's clear we need advice. Dr Shackleton's not in the surgery, so we have to wait for the duty doctor to ring us. He suggests we come in, or alternatively call the paramedics. Plan A is impossible, and so, for the first time in her life, Jane dials 999. At this point Paul, our son in Manchester, telephones about a possible visit. The implications of the injury are beginning to dawn on us. I can't stand unaided; I can't walk, let alone go up the stairs; I can't get into the toilet; I won't be able to use the car. And we have no idea what's wrong or how long healing will take. Consequently, Paul's on the receiving end of an overwrought phone call. Unknown to us, he contacts others in the family who are nearer to us. Then the ambulance comes from Oxford. The lead paramedic examines me, reckons there are no broken bones and advises alternating painkillers. If we are still worried at the weekend, we should have it looked at again.

That was how I had my first taste of acute and disabling pain added to the regular diet of MND, and it reduced me to tears. It was not only the pain, though I discovered I was less stoical than I imagined; it was also the accumulated nights of interrupted sleep and increasing tiredness. I loathed the nights that separated us, as I now slept in my study, while Jane was up in our bedroom. We had to borrow a commode, and even so I couldn't clean myself afterwards. All the everyday operations of life – washing, eating, drinking, getting around – became difficult. And as the tiredness built up, so my voice became less distinct and the muscles round the shoulder tightened and ached. I was not a good patient, even though I had reason to be grateful. By the Sunday it was clear there had not been an improvement, but the four-monthly visit from Lesley, my physio, just happened to be due on the Monday. She ordered me to the Minor Injuries Unit in Abingdon Hospital, where she has her base. Our friend Dan, whose wife has been disabled for many years, gave us a lift in their roll-on-roll-off vehicle. There was the usual Monday morning backlog, but it was not long before I was summoned through to the nurse practitioner. After a combined examination by nurse and physio, my shoulder was x-rayed and tissue damage only diagnosed. At the same time Lesley ordered a commode, a holding belt and a hospital bed, which were delivered to our home in little more than twenty-four hours. Again, for me the system was amazingly efficient.

The hospital bed, which could be raised and lowered electrically, provided the most immediate relief. Before its arrival, I had used our light spare bed, which was low and necessitated both Jane and Bryan (who had come home to help) to get me into and out of it, with a degree of histrionics on my part. With the hospital bed set at the right height, Jane was able to do it on her own and Bryan could go back to begin his new job. But it would be weeks before I was capable of getting up the stairs again, to sleep with my wife in our comfortable bed.

So, also, I learned an instant lesson in helplessness and dependence. I had thought I was coping reasonably well with the slowly rising tide, but this was like being dropped overboard out of sight of land – and I'm not a good swimmer. I tend to panic when my head goes under water. Etched on my memory is swimming alone in the pool of a French campsite. Suddenly cramp seized my right leg, and for a few moments I floundered in a cold sweat (or its water-borne equivalent) towards my depth. I never swam alone again.

Now I was suddenly out of my depth once more. Any movement of my right arm sent shooting pains deep into my shoulder, it seemed. For some weeks I could put no weight on it, and it became clear that, if I was not careful, I would keep aggravating the injury and risk it becoming permanent. Lesley, the physiotherapist, issued dire warnings, and for once I tried to follow her instructions to the letter. I avoided actions that were painful. This meant I could not use the toilet, and got accustomed to using the calabash-shaped plastic urinal, with its oddly inscribed blue lid – 'Do not exceed 70°C' – which stretched the imagination. Wouldn't you be dead if your pee was coming out that hot? Then there was the commode, and Jane having to clean my backside. I know it's commonplace for carers, but even so, it seemed a demeaning task for one's wife.

Settling for the night downstairs became a routine. My muscles would tighten up as the evening wore on, and I would have to balance the increasing discomfort against long restless nights. Physically getting to bed was a juggling act, as well. With limited space next to the bed, we eventually worked out the optimum order of operations to tip my uncooperative carcass out of the wheelchair and on and into the bed. And so, kissed goodnight like a child, I would lie there in the dark, on my back, waiting for friendly sleep. Usually I was so tired that I would soon be asleep.

In a few hours, however, wakefulness would arrive, heralded by some odd dreams echoing the radio if I'd failed to set the 'Sleep' button, and exposing an aching shoulder, or back, or sore heels. Lying there in the dark, I experienced real helplessness. I could reach the bedside table with my left hand, but shifting position was impossible. My last and only resort was to ring Jane's number on the mobile, waken her and bring her down to help, which naturally I was reluctant to do. It was enough each evening to see the exhaustion and pain etched on her face, as she stood by my bedside, after the struggle of helping me to bed. It felt as if I could see her aging before my eyes.

One night, in the dead hours, I woke up more uncomfortable than ever: shoulder, bladder and back were all yelling. What little shuffling I could do made no difference. I would not last the night. So I reached for the mobile. It was tuned in to Jane's number. I pressed the send button – and the light went out. Well, I thought, perhaps the signal's been sent. After a few minutes and no sign of Jane, I tried again. The light came on; I pressed send, and it died. The battery had run down. The door was shut. Vicarages are often designed so that the work area, the 'study', is isolated from the rest of the house, for the privacy of visitors and for the convenience of any family living at home. Ours conforms to the pattern, as I proved. I shouted. I shouted in bursts. I shouted louder. I didn't know I could still shout so loud. There was a filing cabinet by my head. I hit it repeatedly with my mobile phone. If it ruined my phone, I didn't care. But there was neither sign nor sound of life stirring in the rest of the house. The dog didn't even bother to bark. I tried shouting again. 'Hello-o ... hello-o ... hello...' It suddenly occurred to me, 'This is the sound we hear at night from the nursing home.' The plaintive, frustrated, desperate cry of helplessness. In the end, I gave up and turned on the radio. Dozing fitfully, I waited for the morning, and for Jane to come down to let the chickens and the dog out. When she reached me, I was less than gracious in my welcome – but I was relieved to see her. It had been a long night.

The days, too, were long and unproductive. Sitting still produced new aches and pains in my back. My skin dried out and became flaky. Jane washed my hair in a bowl. I kept changes of clothes to a minimum, sleeping in my shirt as removing it hurt so much. I left the house only to get to the nearest church at the weekend. At a stroke, my existence was restricted. I felt more useless than ever.

Over the weeks the shoulder healed, the pain lessened, and I was more or less able to return to my former level of normality. Nevertheless, I realized that I had been given a taste of things to come. And I did not relish it. And thus the waiting continues.

Chapter Thirty

They Also Live

I guess waiting is what all of us who have terminal illness do. However much we manage to prolong our active life, all the time the alarm clock ticks away and we wait to hear, 'Your time's up, Michael Wenham!' Or just, remotely, possibly, 'They've found a cure.' But there is waiting, and waiting. It could be that we will sit, huddled and irritable, like passengers in a haunted waiting room, wondering when our train will arrive to take us into the unknown darkness; or we could seize, however painfully, every hour as a reprieve to be grateful for and every day as a new day to live, until our call comes. In the meantime they – the doctors and researchers – explore every avenue in the hunt, and we, the patients, have to be just that ... patient. And our carers have perhaps the hardest job: living with the unpredictable, knowing only that our condition will get worse, their burden will get heavier, and in the end they will be left with mere memories.

At this point, while I'm still able to, I want to invest in a bank of good memories – days out, holidays, family celebrations, evenings coming together by the fire, revisiting former haunts, rekindling old passions, but also discovering new ones. So it's not just waiting. It is living. Life goes on. In

2007 three posters appeared on the London underground. The caption on one reads: 'Rosie was diagnosed with the fatal disease MND. She has just been found floating down the river.' The picture shows Rosie Fraser, aged 44, at the helm of a sailing dinghy. The next caption reads: 'Brian was diagnosed with the fatal disease MND. He recently went out and bought a gun.' The picture shows Brian Wells, who's 60, on his electric scooter playing with a water pistol with his grandchildren. The third caption reads: 'Esther was diagnosed with the fatal disease MND. She has just been found with a needle in her arm.' The picture shows Esther, a 33-year-old mother, being tattooed on her arm.

To meet them or to read their blogs, it is clear that life isn't easy; it isn't all fun and games. As we wait, the strain tells. The depending irks. I don't like Jane having to live her life round my needs, not being able to go out until she has dressed me, having to come back to make me lunch, not being able to go to bed until I have dragged myself reluctantly upstairs, having to put toothpaste on the brush for me, having to undress me before she can lie down and get some sleep at last. Although I know she does it gladly and wouldn't want it otherwise, I can't believe that sometimes she doesn't resent it – the disease rather than me. And I would certainly want it otherwise. I wish she didn't have to do all the considerable gardening herself, all the driving, shopping, cooking, all the physical work. I wish ... I wish... It sounds like a children's game, but this is real enough. Becoming more and more limited is an acute affliction: the horizon closing in, immobility marching closer, silence falling on vocal cords, 'eating' through a tube, suffocating from inside, helpless to help yourself... And yet life goes on, and with it a defiant assertion, 'I won't allow the glaring headlights of fear on the road ahead to paralyse me. I am not a rabbit. I am a human being of infinite worth, up to and beyond my final breath. I want to be remembered that way.'

The art of dying – we need to think and talk more about it. Death is the last enemy. It's also the last taboo. John Donne defied it as 'one short sleep past';[1] Dylan Thomas raged at it as 'the dying of the light', while his father lay on his deathbed.[2] When Damien Hirst encrusted a skull with diamonds and put it on the art market for $100 million, he asserted he was 'definitely giving the V to death'. I wouldn't put it like that; but the real worthwhile art is to celebrate our life as long as we have it and simultaneously to accept the fact of our mortality. There are few sadder spectacles than rich people hoping to trick death through cryogenics. Life is the first gift we receive – for better or worse. But it has an expiry date. My view is that we are no more responsible for when it ends than for when it begins. What we *are* uniquely responsible for is what we do with it in the interim. I don't believe in ineluctable fate, a blind predetermining of when we are born and when we die; but I believe that those end points of our existence are outside of our proper competencies. However, in the meantime, we are to make the most of what we are given. For example, after my diagnosis, I ceased to take each day for granted. I would wake up and think, with something like elation, 'Thank God, I'm alive to see another day.' I hope I will continue to feel the same, even as the disease ruthlessly restricts my life bit by bit. Yet equally I hope that, when the time comes, whether it's a struggle or not, I'll be able to accept that life was given, life was full and life has been taken away.

This book is being finished in the memory of someone intimately involved in our story. Rosemary was Jane's chief bridesmaid at our wedding. Her husband, John, was my best man. Two years ago Rosemary, who was a nurse and mother, was diagnosed with aggressive bowel cancer. She had radical surgery and violent chemotherapy, which delayed but did not prevent it from spreading. Of course, Rosemary was all too aware of the critical nature of her condition, but there was no way that she would allow it to subdue her. She holidayed on the continent, went skiing, paragliding and swimming. She continued working, and would cycle up Headington Hill to her hospital appointments in Oxford. Even when she knew she had entered the 'end game', she planned expeditions, played tennis and travelled to visit family. At 4.30am on 1 May her family picked her up from Michael Sobell House, the hospice where she was receiving treatment, and punted her up the river to hear the choristers sing in May Morning at Magdalen Bridge. Later she had one more outing on the river. On 12 May 2007 she died in the hospice, while the sun broke through the clouds.

She left a message for her friends and family. It was read at her memorial service. In it she reflected on dying:

> Strive to live each day as if it's your last because we don't know when death will come. It's a fact of life that, as we are born, so we will die, and without being morbid it's a useful idea to hold on to, even if lightly – so let's try and face mortality with equanimity. A possibly appropriate attitude with which to die is not necessarily with fortitude, but with trust and final surrender... Don't be too sad. We plan for a good birth for our children. Let's also plan for a good death for ourselves.

That is making the most of the meantime.

Notes

[1] John Donne, Holy Sonnet 3.

[2] In the poem 'Do not go gentle into that good night'.

Afterword

What is MND?

I have inevitably written about motor neurone disease, since it's the condition I know best, but I hope that others with similarly degenerative diseases will recognize similarities with their own experience. It occurs to me, however, that MND is relatively rare, affecting only about 5,000 at any one time in this country, and some sort of description might be useful.

I am not a doctor or a scientist, and so what follows is very much a layman's understanding of the condition, or more accurately conditions, known as motor neurone disease in the UK. Elsewhere it's called amyotrophic lateral sclerosis (ALS: see below). In the United States it's known as Lou Gehrig's disease, after the great New York Yankees baseball player, who died from it on 2 June 1941.

The motor neurones (or, more trendily, neurons) are the cells which transmit instructions from the brain to the muscles. MND is the umbrella term used in the UK for conditions when the motor neurons are damaged. Unlike cancer, in which cells grow out of control, in MND they deteriorate out of control, and in an adult these cells can't replace themselves. It's like links in a communication system going down and having no engineer able to repair them. For a time you may manage to get round the problem, but bit by bit more links go down, until eventually the whole system shuts down – all but the control centre, which is the brain.

At that point you have no choice but to haul up the white flag and admit defeat, or, if you prefer, pack up and go home.

The form of MND depends partly on which motor neurones are affected: either upper (from the brain to the spinal cord) or lower (from the spine to the muscles round the body). The commonest form, affecting about two-thirds of us, is amyotrophic lateral sclerosis (ALS). In this both upper and lower motor neurones are damaged. The next most common is progressive bulbar palsy (PBP), affecting about a quarter of us, where the damage is first to the head and neck. These two are the most aggressive forms. About 10 per cent of cases are progressive muscular atrophy (PMA), where the lower motor neurones are damaged and onset tends to be younger than in other forms. The rarest form, in which the damage is to the upper motor neurones, is primary lateral sclerosis (PLS), which is my diagnosis.

A question the doctors ask you is, 'Has anyone else in your family had MND?' In 90–95 per cent of cases the answer is no, but 5–10 per cent of cases are 'familial': that is, there is a genetic factor involved. Although the symptoms are indistinguishable between familial and sporadic MND, clearly it is easier to research genetic strains than those which have no obvious links. At the moment, there is no known cause for MND. Most research is focused on trying to uncover a cause, or causes, on the grounds that, when you know that, you can more effectively target treatment and even prevention. Research is highlighting possible factors, but there's been no acclaimed breakthrough yet. The fact that life expectancy is short with MND poses acute problems for research into and trialling of treatments. In fact there's only one drug routinely prescribed for MND, riluzole, which can extend life expectancy for a few months. I'm not taking it myself, having decided it wasn't worth it for me.

However, as I hope this book shows, I do benefit from the care that's provided both by the National Health Service and voluntarily. In some ways this is more costly, in terms of personal investment, than prescribing a pill, but it is, in my opinion, of the greatest value. It involves sharing pain and exposing oneself to loss. When it is willingly given, rather than granted as a right, I have a feeling that it is more than therapeutic. I reckon it transforms a lonely dark journey into an experience of the best of humanity. It may even be redemptive.

For More Information

The MNDA provides a great deal of accessible and comprehensible information, for example on its website. For those who want to understand the condition better, I recommend it as the first port of call (www.mndassociation.org). The US equivalent is the ALSA (www.alsa.org).

Back Cover Material

The story of a church minister's struggle with Motor Neurone or Lou Gehrig's Disease, told with courage, humour and faith.

It began with a slight unsteadiness. After months of tests at the Radcliffe Infirmary in Oxford, the consultant said, 'Revd Wenham, would you like to sit down?' Michael, who had helped so many through terminal illness, now faced his own sentence. Would his faith stand the heat?

'His brilliant story-telling makes the book hard to put down; his gentle humour delights and warms the reader ... I love this book. I think you will too.'

–Elaine Storkey, president of Tearfund and broadcaster

'A beautifully written, honest story about suffering and grace.'

–Simon Ponsonby, writer and theologian

'No glib answers, no false comfort, just a joyful, humbling, funny and very realistic account ... very inspiring.'

–Stephen Cottrell, Bishop of Reading

'Gives the ammunition to fight back and the courage to confront head-on any terminal disease. It is a must-read for those facing such a diagnosis, their families and friends.'

–Jean Waters, trustee of the Motor Neurone Disease Association, and herself a sufferer from MND

Made in United States
Cleveland, OH
05 November 2026

47668297R00108